# LOW BACK PAIN

relieve    recondition

# P R O G R A M

## Instructional TRAINING Guide

*effective targeted exercises* for *long term pain relief*

13 MOBILITY exercises FOR PAIN RELIEF
19 PROGRESSIVE exercises TO RECONDITION
13 CHALLENGE exercises FOR PREVENTION
10 MAINTENANCE exercises TO PROTECT

45 Exercises, Movements and Stretches
170 Detailed Illustrations

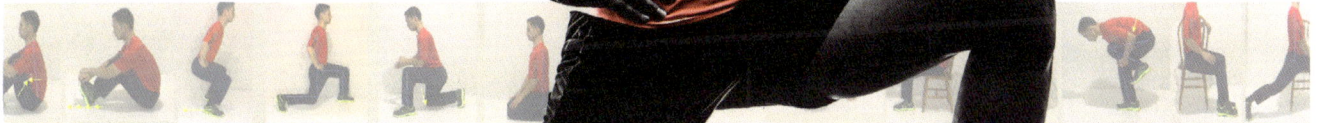

An Easy, Step-by-Step, Safe, Self-Treatment Plan to Help Reduce Your Need for Medication or Surgery

4 Treatment Levels
4 Progress Charts

## SHERWIN NICHOLSON Hon. B.Sc.

lowbackpainprogram.com

SN HEALTH RESOURCES

L O N G   T E R M   R E L I E F - N O T   P A I N

# Low Back Pain Program

ISBN 978-0-9937737-0-9 (ebook)

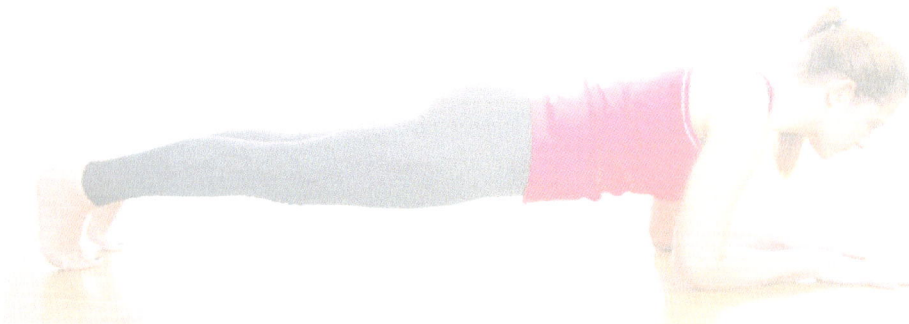

# Contents

# Part One - What to Know

## Introduction - A word from the Author

First and foremost, thank you for your interest and for purchasing the E-book. It will prove to be of great benefit and an important tool toward your commitment to resolving long term lower back pain. This book will help you to progress from a life of daily discomfort, limitations and frustration from your lower back pain issues, to one with increasing mobility, pain relief and freedom. It requires your commitment and hard work and will be worth the time, effort and patience required.

I personally understand the struggle that you have with this very serious issue. It is probably one of the most debilitating conditions to have and takes both a physical and emotional toll on you. It is not just the struggle of having the pain, but also the frustration and disappointment that comes with believing that your pain has been reduced or resolved later in the day, week, etc.. only to return again. Sometimes, this cycle of pain and the effects that it has on us actually feels more painful that the pain in our lower back.

I have helped many that have had similar issues with their lower back and have provided them with the relief that they have needed. Because I have had this problem myself and struggled with it for more than 10 years, I truly know the struggle that you have now. It is simply one of the most unfair and silent problems that one can ever experience.

You have my full understanding, compassion and devotion for your lower back pain relief. I wish your pain could simply end immediately without the need for any E-book at all. However, the book is meant to teach you the skills and exercises that will help you come out of your struggle. This is why I am compelled to help others, create the website and book.

In order to succeed with using this book, you must read it in its entirety and not skip to the exercises. By reading everything in the book before beginning, you will be able to understand why each exercise is required and what it means to perform it. You can have a better mental picture and focus on the muscle groups and joints involved and learn how to target and engage them each time that you use them.

Even though I know your struggle, I cannot begin to know all of the issues associated with your lower back pain. Hopefully that is between you and your medical doctor. The complexity of your lower back pain will certainly affect the success of this program for you. I cannot guarantee a complete recovery by using this program because of the complexity of lower back pain and your personal commitment to it. I can assure you that what I have written in this book is essential for your long term health and relief of lower back pain associated with your back muscles and joints. Regardless of the extent of your back pain, you will benefit from the exercises.

I wish you the best possible recovery for your lower back pain and new possibilities for a pain free lifestyle.

Truly,

Sherwin.

## Lower Back Pain Issues

Lower back pain can result from a wide range of issues. Direct or indirect physical injury to the spine. Aging, disease or genetic factors. Acute or chronic overuse and underuse of the muscles that support and protect the spine. Even a combination of these can be present, which is more likely to be the case.

Some of these issues require simple rest and time while some require more serious medical attention well beyond the scope and information provided by this book. This book is intended to provide information to address the pain in the lower back resulting from muscular imbalances. These imbalances are occurring as a result of chronic over and underuse of the muscles that support and protect the lumbar spine.

This chronic condition causes imbalances to occur in the various layers of muscle that keep the spine stable. Imbalances lead to poor distribution of pressure along the edges of the lumbar vertebrae and spinal discs. Excessive pressure can lead to disc failure and pressure on the nerves that travel along the spine. A combination of these events can lead to a range of problems ranging from back fatigue, back spasm, lumbar disc bulge, herniated lumbar disc, vertebral damage, mild to severe nerve pain or back muscle pain, and also pain downstream from the spine to the lower limbs.

*If you have suffered a serious injury directly to the discs or spine (such as a fall or accident), medical attention is required first as it can be dangerous to exercise while injured. Follow the advice of your doctor first and then ask for consent prior to beginning this program.*

When these issues become chronic and adequate treatment is not pursued, it becomes progressively more risky to the long term health of the spine.

Low back pain can impact day to day functioning in the following areas: an inability to sleep well, stand or sit for long periods of time, lift or carry heavy or awkward objects, perform hobbies or sports for any significant amount of time, perform well while working on the job, simply enjoy life without the fatigue and stress, or having constant pain - to name a few. These issues are serious because they affect our quality of life and relationships.

What is common with all of these issues is that your lower back muscles, hip and leg muscles, and to some degree other areas of your body, must perform correctly in order for *any* of these groups to function properly and to protect your back. The very muscles themselves that may not be functioning properly will also exhibit chronic pain that you may interpret as lower back pain. By improving their functioning, the pain produced by them will also subside.

You can get help to relieve these issues through the Low Back Pain Program, an exercise program which is designed to target these areas.

## The Proper Mindset

A successful exercise program to help relieve lower back pain must be comprehensive but honest. The truth about this program is that it will require much time and effort. Possibly more than you may expect. Why? Because the long road that leads us to chronic low back pain is one that we may simply believe may have come on suddenly, but it simply hasn't. Having a painless back one day and then a painful one the next day may seem sudden. What has not changed is the underlying issues that caused your back to 'give out' that next day. It was there for a long time, when you felt that your back was 'fine'.
A misunderstanding of the problem, or lack of awareness of it occurred and consequently, resulted in treating the symptoms with medication or rest. You may have thought that your pain was the result of fatigue. However your body is sending you subtle signals that something requires attention and not merely pampering.

*Do not misinterpret body pain as something to be avoided but as something to listen to. A warning sign.*

When you lean over to pick up an object, and your body does not engage its muscles or joints in the correct order, strength or position, something else will overcompensate to perform the task.

There is no free lunch when it comes to body mechanics. The body part that is overcompensating will painfully react, informing you that you moved incorrectly. This pain is understood as a signal from your body to engage the other muscle groups more actively.

In time you will learn to respond to the needs of your body and engage the correct muscles at the right time. The time that you will need to learn this will be extensive as there are many muscular groups and joints that will be asked to move and function differently than before. Some muscles and joints have been immobile, tight, stiff, weak and even non responsive when called in to action. Training these muscles to function again will be challenging as you know that they will be in use often and for longer times than before.

You will feel sore and tired as with any exercise or workout program. However these muscles are the very ones that have been reacting and complaining all along. This time, they will not be sending pain signals from abuse or overcompensation, but instead they will be put to proper use and conditioning.

Unfortunately, you may still interpret the discomfort as lower back pain and believe that you are not making progress as the pain is 'still there'. Be patient and persist as this is the signal that your body is sore or tired from exercise and not from overuse or strain. This mindset matters as you will be able to know the differences and meet the challenges or demands on your body better than before.

Think of the problems associated with back pain as layers of an onion with respect to your muscles and joints involved. As you peel and remove one layer (problem), another layer just as thick but deeper is uncovered. Some of us get stuck peeling that top layer or two off, only to put them back on later. It feels like an endless cycle and leads to frustration and dissatisfaction with rehabilitation. We quit. Each layer requires persistence, and with lower back pain, there are many layers to peel before long term relief is acheived.

Back pain is not simply one general area of pain but a culmination over time of many smaller sources of pain that combine and amplify. You are not really trying to eliminate one source but slowly isolate, treat and relieve many individual ones. That is why you don't get instant relief or why it feels like there is little progress. Don't be confused or discouraged by pain and what it may signify: As one set of muscles becomes better conditioned, another weaker set gets recruited but will surely complain about it. This is an example of pain that signifies progress.

The program has specific exercises to address the different 'layers' you will peel. You will begin with the most gentle methods and progress to more challenging ones. After these exercises, you can then maintain your back with a smaller, select group of the exercises.

Recovery time is also according to the complexities specific to *your* back pain. You will progress according to the needs of your body. The lifestyle and actions that led you to the pain that you have and the unique abilities of your body are different from anyone else; your body will tell you when you will recover. Don't just look for relief, look for progress, and progress takes time.

Most of us enjoy being physically active, but that is when our bodies are physically comfortable. Very few of us actually like to engage in any type of intense exercise or training when there is likelihood for strain or discomfort. We just don't see the benefit, so we avoid it.

It is understandable that we would want to avoid this kind of situation, however I believe that this is not a sufficient reason for quitting: The exercises in this book are not the type that you should avoid, as they are meant to protect the body. It can be seen as a waste of time to pick up something very heavy repeatedly if it will only make you look good in the mirror. It can also be seen as a waste of time to persist in a sport while your body is suffering pain from an imbalance as described earlier. You may have other examples yourself. I ask that you see these exercises as movements that your body needs despite some discomfort as you progress.

I hope that this has been helpful in establishing the proper mindset in order to begin the Low Back Pain Program. You will be challenged but it will be well worth the effort and time.

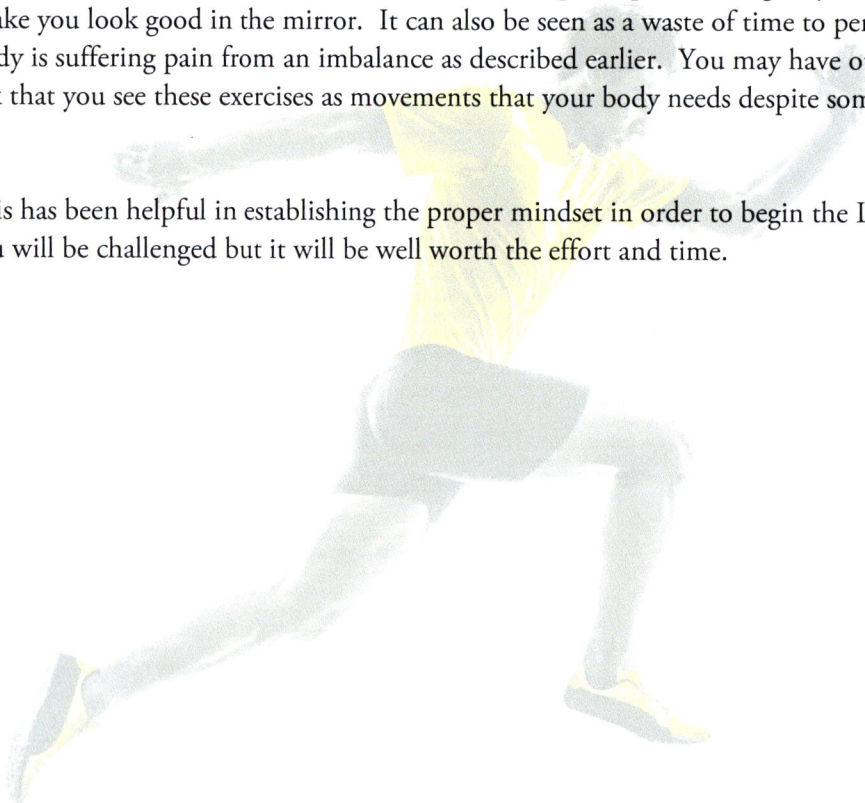

## Program Preparation

Back pain has many different causes so there is likely an extensive amount of treatment required. The amount of time that you will need for each exercise will also be extensive. In time, when the target areas have improved, you will no longer need the same amount of time to condition each muscle group. The muscles and joints will be more responsive, stronger and stable and you will move through the exercises faster and should be able to omit some of them later as you progress.

You do not need a lot of space or any equipment. Dress comfortably so that your hips are not restricted by your clothing. Jeans are not advised as they restrict the opening of the hips and are counter to flexibility. Non-slip footwear or bare feet is safer. Have a soft carpet, padded floor, chair, bed or couch available for stability and comfort. Avoid distractions such as phones or gadgets until later, after you have progressed past the initial exercises. Some exercises require a padded floor to protect the knees or seat while some require the bare floor for balance. *Some pictures are illustrated with arrows and axis lines to provide a guide for correct positioning of your spine, hips and legs. Blue lines indicate your required spine, pelvis, hip and leg positions while yellow arrows indicate movements, contractions and stretches.*

Many of the exercises, movements and stretches can be done anytime and anywhere. Wherever and whenever you find the opportunity to perform them, do. You can make the most of your time with the program if you blend the exercises in with other activities. Many can be done while watching television, in bed and at the same time as other activities as they are functional exercises.

Allow yourself to breath slowly and deeply. It will help you to relax throughout the exercises. Many exercises may bring some discomfort as you begin to mobilize and lengthen very tight muscles and joints. Careful and controlled breaths will help as your tension gradually decreases.

Finally, it may be easy to become overwhelmed by all of the exercises. Be patient. You know your own limitations. Take your time. Do what you can and with the time available, but try to cover all of them. By doing this, you are tackling the problem from different angles. You are trying to rebuild years of lost strength and imbalances that have developed slowly over time. If it takes longer than you thought, it is OK. This is your time, and your body. You will be making progress with each exercise.

I encourage you to be vigilant in learning about your body, the muscle groups involved, the joints affected and what their day-to-day needs are. By doing so, you will regain an ability to better enjoy a body conscious, productive and satisfying personal and work life.

*The information on the Low Back Pain Program website will help provide more understanding of the different areas of the body that specifically affect the lower back. You can read the information available on the site and of course many other sites to enrich your background knowledge. You can find the information by clicking the 'back pain' button found on the categories bar on the page. The website explains vital information about the 'core', the lumbar spine, vertebral discs, back muscles and abdominals, hip flexors and hamstrings, acute and chronic pain, lifestyle, exercise, treatment and prevention, and finally, the importance of dedicating time for effective stretching.*

# Part Two - What to Do

## The Low Back Pain Program Exercise Outline

The exercises in the program are to be performed in a step by step, progressive order. They are divided into five categories. Categories 1 through 4 cover the different stages that your body will perform at and progress through and are specific to the program. Category 5 provides a list of supportive exercises that are available from many other common sources beneficial to the program.

The first category takes into account the limited mobility, strength, range of motion, flexibility and discomfort that you may have prior to beginning. As you improve in one category you will be able to move on to the next one. It is important to cover all areas required in each category but you do not have to complete every exercise before moving on to the next category. However, it is advisable to return periodically to complete the unfinished exercises to benefit fully from the program.

## Limited Mobility Exercises

- To relieve tension and lengthen tight muscles and joints.
- To re-align joints, improve range of motion and stimulate flexibility.
- Significant time is required to progress well in this level. It is very important to accomplish these introductory exercises. Once mastered, you will not be required to perform them anymore unless tightness returns.

## Progressive Exercises

- To strengthen weakened muscles, add stability to unstable muscles groups, reinstate flexibility.
- Create more mobility in resistant muscles and to rebalance muscles and joints.
- This level requires more strength training and balance.
- These exercise are numerous but important to perform as they involve a multidirectional approach to addressing your lower back issues.
- In time, you will only need to perform these exercises as needed.

## Challenging Exercises

- To improve stability, balance, strength at longer durations.
- To create more endurance to reduce fatigue and improve stamina.
- This level requires the most effort and balance of all categories.
- These exercises, although not easy, will become easier with more mobility, strength and balance.
- You may want to perform these occasionally after some extensive time of training.

## Maintenance Exercises

♦ To condition the muscles to perform and function effectively with more complex movements and tasks.

♦ This level requires the least amount of time but the most effort in execution. These exercises are to be done weekly. You will find it easy to perform in between and with your everyday movements as they are intended to be functional and practical.

## Supportive Exercises

♦ These exercises are familiar and beneficial exercises for overall lower back pain treatment.

♦ They can be performed at any time and in any amount within your comfort level.

♦ I do not go into detail about how to perform these exercises as they can be learned from other sources.

With respect to the program exercises, *I do not recommend a specific number of repetitions. Repetition quantity is secondary in priority to the degree of progress, mobility and strengthening that you are making. Whether you choose to perform 5 repetitions or 20 should depend on your comfort level.* The number of repetitions that we choose should be on an individual basis. At the end of each exercise, use your own discretion according to your comfort level to determine how often you would like to repeat each exercise, as long as you can perform them properly and effectively before moving on to a more difficult one. There may be times when you are able to perform an exercise with many repetitions well, but then with only a few repetitions at another time. Do not skip any exercises or perform them quickly. Do them carefully, slowly, and often.

*When you initially begin to stretch, your muscles will react by tightening up to resist the stretch. It will take anywhere from 10 seconds to 2 full minutes for the muscle to relax and no longer resist the stretch. After that time period, your muscle will be more cooperative and will lengthen. This is the time when your stretch is most effective and productive. You will develop a sense of when your muscle is responding to your stretch and your muscle will respond faster over the weeks to come. Be vigilant not to stop your stretch period prematurely.*

Part Three of the book provides a set of charts that list each exercise for categories 1 through 4. Complete the charts according to your own level of comfort and not by repetition of exercises. When you can perform an exercise easily and comfortably, with little or no pain and for a reasonable duration of time, you should progress on to the next exercise.

## Limited Mobility Exercises

Deep Squat Rest
Kneeling Bow Rest
Seated Leg Opener
Seated Leg Rotation (assisted)
Seated Twist (assisted)
Seated Lunge
Leg Stretch (hamstrings and quads)
Calf Stretch
Hangs and Pushes
Lying Twist
Abdominal Crunch
Quadriceps Stretch
Seated Knee Raise

## Progressive Exercises

Seated Hip Adjustment (assisted)
Seated and Floor Hip Shift
Seated Leg Rotation (assisted with contraction)
Seated Leg Cross with Forward Lean
Floor Leg Bend and Shift
Seated Leg to Chest
Leaning Hip Shift
Rail Squat (assisted)
Seated Hamstring Stretch
Stair Step (up and down)
Reverse Stair Squat Lean
Hip Opener (inside and outside)
Seated Calf Stretch
Double Leg Rotation
Deep Abdominal Crunch (leg raised)
Plank with Steps
Couch Split
Outside Hip Stretch
Standing Abdominal

## Challenging Exercises

Seated Leg Lift (multidirectional)
Advanced Hamstring Stretch (ankle and floor)
Squat (holds, leans, circles, steps, walks)
Lunge with Reverse Kneel
Reverse Lunge
Reverse Stair Step
Standing Knee to Chest (upright and leaning)
Standing Hip Shift (leaning and bent knee)
Forward Stair Step with Hip Shift (assisted 2 riser)
Standing Leg Raise with Side Kick
Leg Flex (rail or counter)
Foot Raise (lean and bend)
Abdominal Leg Press

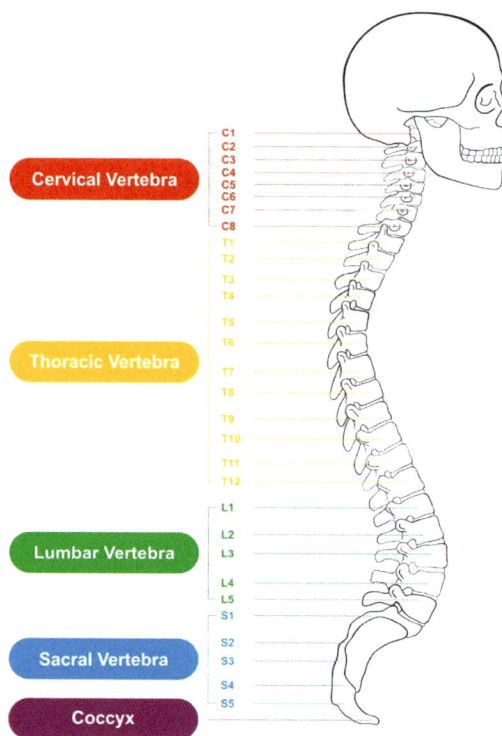

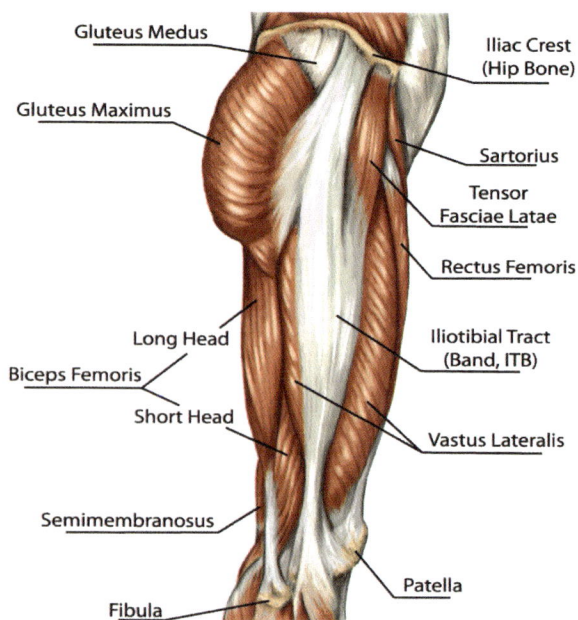

8

## Maintenance Exercises

Squat (walks)
Abdominal Leg Press
Seated Leg Rotation
Standing Abdominals
Plank with Steps
Lunge with Reverse Kneel
Foot Raise (leaning and bent knee)
Advanced Hamstring Stretch
Forward Stair Step with Hip Shift
Reverse Lunge

## Supportive exercises

standing hamstring stretch
seated leg fold
side splits
side lean
lying rotator stretch
abdominal stretch (cobra)
floor hip stretch
buttock stretch (lying or standing)
balancing quad stretch
bridges

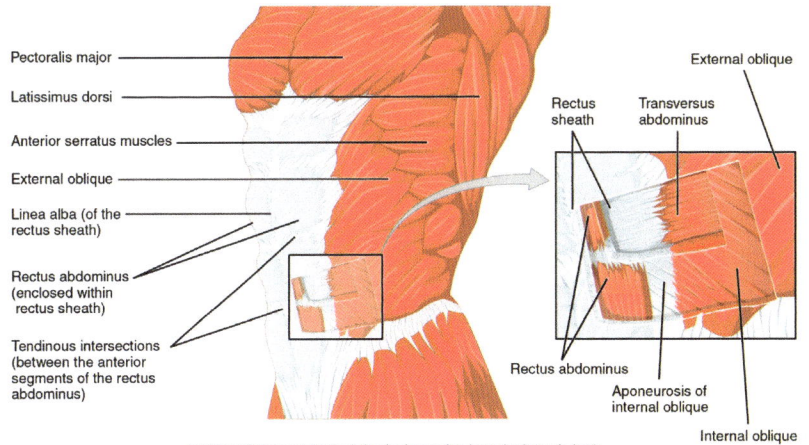

Pectoralis major
Latissimus dorsi
Anterior serratus muscles
External oblique
Linea alba (of the rectus sheath)
Rectus abdominus (enclosed within rectus sheath)
Tendinous intersections (between the anterior segments of the rectus abdominus)

External oblique
Rectus sheath
Transversus abdominus
Rectus abdominus
Aponeurosis of internal oblique
Internal oblique

(a) Superficial and deep abdominal muscles (anterior lateral view)

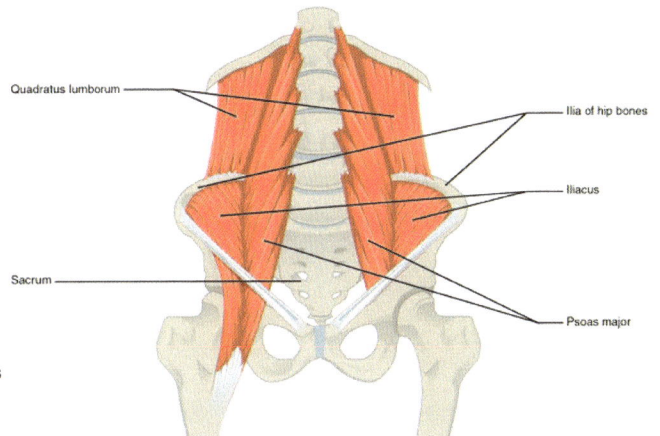

Quadratus lumborum
Sacrum
Ilia of hip bones
Iliacus
Psoas major

(b) Posterior abdominal muscles (anterior view)

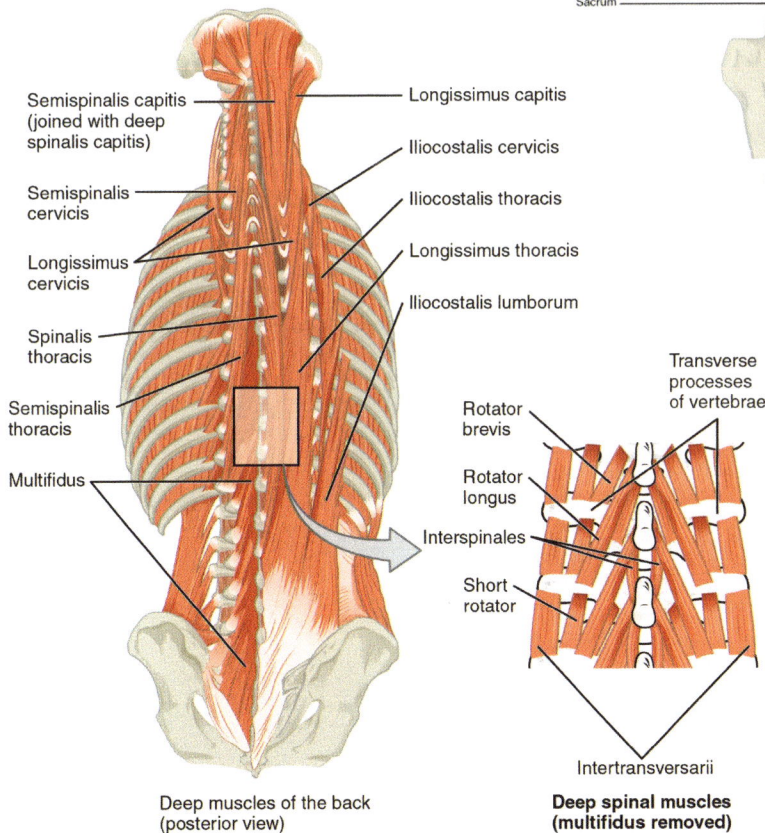

Semispinalis capitis (joined with deep spinalis capitis)
Semispinalis cervicis
Longissimus cervicis
Spinalis thoracis
Semispinalis thoracis
Multifidus

Longissimus capitis
Iliocostalis cervicis
Iliocostalis thoracis
Longissimus thoracis
Iliocostalis lumborum

Deep muscles of the back (posterior view)

Transverse processes of vertebrae
Rotator brevis
Rotator longus
Interspinales
Short rotator
Intertransversarii

**Deep spinal muscles (multifidus removed)**

# Limited Mobility Exercises

## Deep Squat Rest

This exercise will determine how tight your lower back and hips are initially.  Shortened leg and hip muscles may prevent you from resting fully.  You may feel at first that you cannot perform this well, but with more flexibility, it will become easier.  This squat will help to release the tightness in your lower back and help to open up the hip area.  Try to perform this exercise as often as possible initially in order to condition the joints to relax faster each time that you perform it.  The exercise helps to counter anterior pelvic tilt.

Step 1:  Stand upright with feet shoulder width apart.

Step 2:  Slowly lower your body to a full squat position while keeping your upper body vertical.

Step 3:  As you come lower, bring your belly button to your thighs and relax while resting your arms in front.  Your knees and legs should be closed.

Step 4:  Rest in this position for 1 minute or until you feel that your stomach and chest are fully resting on your thighs.

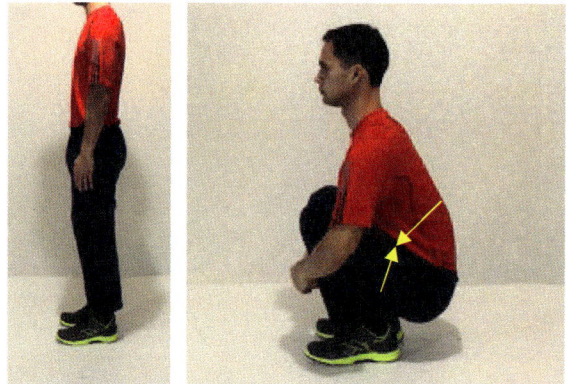

Some of us may find that we are so tight and inflexible that we may lose balance as we do this.  Be patient as your body is not accustomed to being in this position normally.

*Tip:  Hold this position as if you were trying to squeeze a sponge that is in between your belly button and thighs.  Do not force the rest by squeezing your arms around your legs.  You are trying to ease into this position and not pull yourself.  This exercise is helpful for morning stiffness and long periods of standing.*

*Application:  First thing in the morning.  After long periods of standing.*

## Kneeling Bow Rest

This is a variation of the Deep Squat Rest. Some may find it easier on the back. The advantage of the Deep Squat Rest is that it helps with your balance and strengthens the leg muscles. This exercise will also help loosen the tightness in the lower back. It will also help loosen your hips as well and counter anterior pelvic tilt.

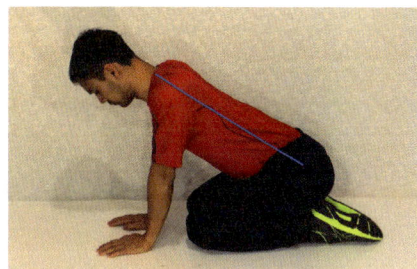

Step 1: Bring yourself down to a kneeling position on both knees while keeping them together. Use soft padding to protect your knees.

Step 2: Sit on your feet and try to contract your stomach muscles.

Step 3: Slowly lean forward starting from the waist and then finally bring your upper chest to your knees.

Step 4: Place your arms out in front and maintain this position for 1 minute or until your stomach is fully rested on your thighs.

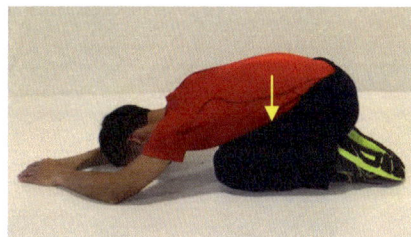

This exercise will take time to perform properly as tightness in the lower back slowly eases. You may need to use your hands to slowly lower your self down in step 3. The goal is to relax and rest in this position and not force it.

*Tip: Hold this position as if you are trying to squeeze a sponge in between your belly button and your thighs. (Use soft padding to protect your knees.) This exercise can be done to help with morning stiffness.*

*Application: After waking while in bed. After long periods of standing.*

## Seated Leg Opener

This exercise stretches your adductors and helps to provide more flexibility in the hips. By loosening tightness in the hip joint, the pelvis has greater range of motion and relieves pressure on the lumbar spine. This exercise is done in the seated position and focuses more on widening the hips than strengthening the legs.

Step 1: Sit comfortably with your back upright and your hands on your knees and feet on the floor

Step 2: With your legs relaxed, use your hands to spread both of your legs slowly outward to the side.

Step 3: When you have opened them as far and as comfortably as they can go, hold this position for 1-2 minutes until tension has subsided.

Step 4: Return to rest position.

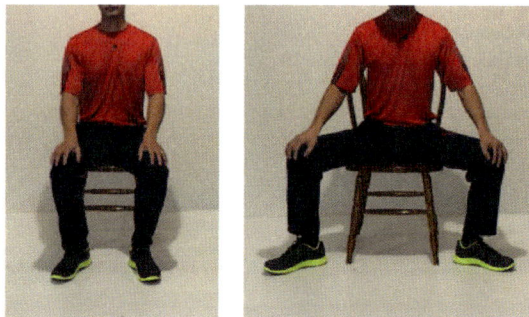

Do not force this stretch. Only use slight pressure to open the legs. Maintain upright posture.

*Tip: It helps to contract the outer muscles of your legs to help widen them, and eventually unassisted by your hands.*

## Seated Leg Rotation (assisted)

This exercise helps to promote greater mobility of your femur. This allows your legs to perform more effectively and to help the pelvis to become more balanced. The normal curvature of your spine will improve. This exercise is done one leg at a time and requires an object such as a book to elevate the feet. You will be using your hands to assist the movement.

Step 1: Sit with your back upright and feet close together. Legs should be bent and at a 90 degree angle.

Step 2: Using a book or a thick cushion, place one foot on the support. Slowly push your knee out as far and as comfortably as possible while keeping your feet together.

Step 3: Hold this position for 1 minute.

Step 4: Repeat this exercise but with the other leg.

Step 5: Start from beginning but with one leg out to the side and foot flat on the ground.

Step 6: Using a book or a thick cushion, again, place one foot on the support. Slowly pull your knee inward toward the other foot while keeping the outward foot motionless. Push as comfortably as you can.

Step 7: Hold this position for 1 minute.

Step 8: Repeat this exercise (from step 6) with the other leg.

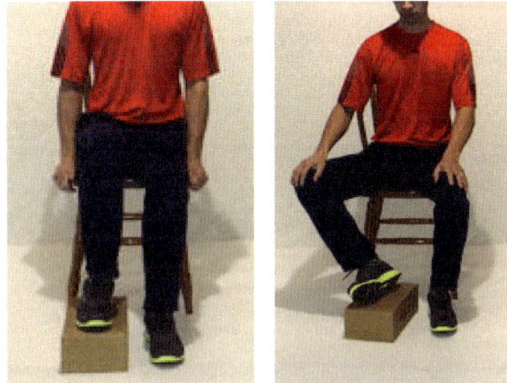

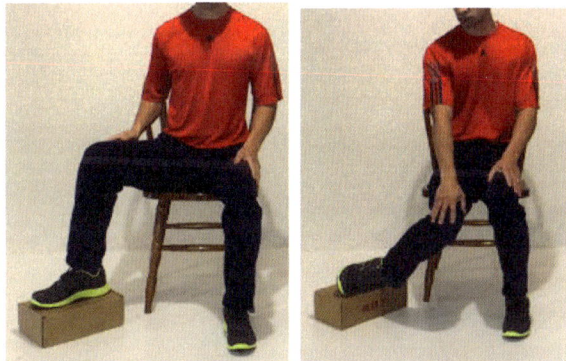

Remember to keep your back upright as you are training for proper posture while using your legs. As you move your knees in and out, you may feel your buttocks lift off the seat slightly. Try to avoid this by relaxing more and using less force.

*Tip: Your 'sit bones' should remain on the seat. The legs should be moving and not the pelvis.*

## Seated Twist (assisted)

It is important to relieve the tension and promote more flexibility in the lower back at this point. Twists are a great way to do this. More freedom with improved twisting with help reduce the number of back spasms associated with reaching for objects beside us. You may find that you are very tight in the lower back and that twisting is very difficult to do. The lumbar vertebrae and muscles do not twist at the same degree as the upper back can. Initially, any twisting accomplished in this exercise will occur in the upper body more than the lower.

The goal is to twist the lower back to mobilize and stretch the muscles. Your back will be tight and resistant at first, but in time, will relax more and you will be able to feel it respond. Your hands should assist you in this exercise.

Step 1: Sit comfortably with knees together and back upright.

Step 2: With one hand beside you and the other behind you, gently rotate your upper body to the side as far and as comfortably as possible.

Step 3: Hold for 1 minute. Rest.

Step 4: Repeat by twisting to the other direction

Step 5: Repeat often.

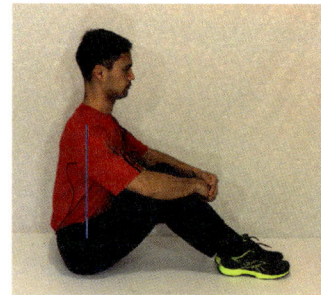

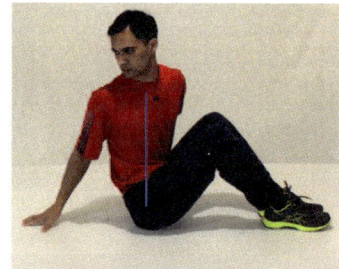

When you are in the hold position, your upper body will respond faster than your lower back. Maintain the hold for a long period of time initially so that the lower back muscles will have a chance to respond. The goal is to relax into a hold and not force a turn. Avoid leaning to the side.

*Tip: When you can perform this exercise easily, do it unassisted without your hands. This allows you to recruit and strengthen the back muscles to actively control your rotational flexibility instead of passively.*

## Seated Lunge

Lunges are normally done without a chair or support. The purpose of the seat is to improve your flexibility and stretch your hip muscles before you execute a full lunge movement. You will need a chair that is stable and/or cushioned. You can position the chair to use the backrest for support. A table will also work. This exercise helps to stretch the psoas muscle. A tight psoas muscle can contribute to low back pain.

**Step 1:** Sit upright with one leg and buttock fully on the seat and the other leg and buttock suspended off of the seat. Keep both knees bent and feet flat.

**Step 2:** With the unsupported leg, slowly slide it to the side and behind you until you are fully stretched out as comfortably as possible. Hold the chair rest or table for stability.

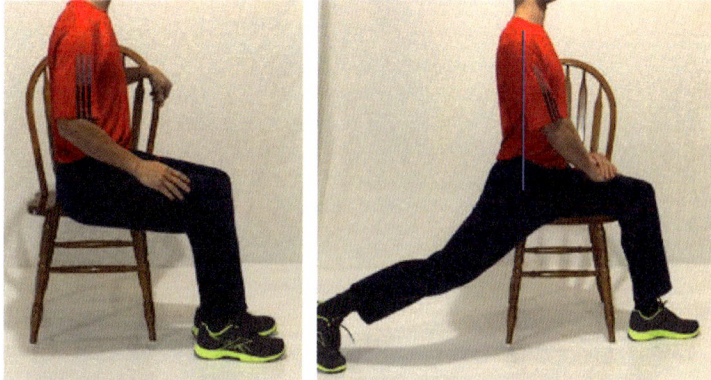

**Step 3:** Try to extend the leg behind you by contracting your thigh muscles and hold this position for 1 minute.

**Step 4:** Repeat this exercise with the other leg.

You may find yourself leaning forward as you extend the leg behind you. Try to avoid this by extending less and maintain an upright posture. Remember, you want to utilize your legs more while your spine is in neutral posture.

*Tip: Contract your abdominals to help counter any excessive anterior pelvic tilt produced from extending your leg behind. This exercise is helpful for when sitting for long periods of time such as at work.*

*Application: Anytime while seated at work or at home.*

## Leg Stretch (hamstrings and quadriceps)

These are your basic passive leg stretches. They do not require any specific instruction. What is important is that although they are basic, they are also fundamental. Even when you do not have back pain, you should be practicing these exercises. Your leg muscles are always in a state of shortening when routinely used. We should stretch them to compensate and balance for it. These exercises can be done anytime and with any stable support. What is important is not to force them but relax into them. Maintain your posture and do take the time to perform them. *Aim for progress each time that you do these, as tight hamstrings and quadriceps are one of the major causes of chronic back pain.*

Step 1: Stand upright and with your back in neutral posture. Using either a chair, table or steps, lift one leg up as high and as comfortably as possible on to the support. You should feel a gentle stretch on the back of your legs.

Step 2: Hold this position for 1-2 minutes minimum.

Step 3: Repeat with the other leg.

Step 4: Stand upright and with your back in neutral posture. While holding onto the support, lift one foot up from behind you and raise the foot to your buttocks. Do this gently. You should feel a gentle stretch on your thigh muscles.

Step 5: Hold this position for 1-2 minutes.

Step 6: Repeat the entire exercise often.

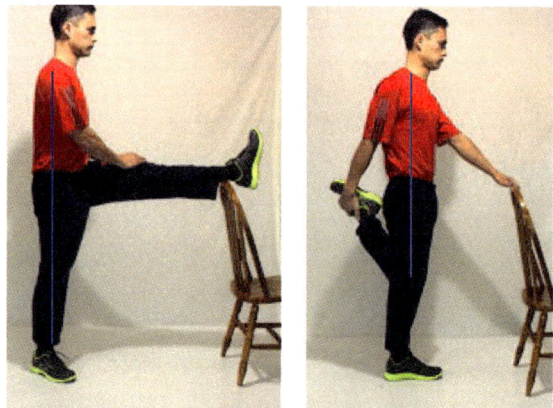

These stretches may not be very comfortable but they are necessary as they will prepare you for more progressive stretches later. It is important to keep your hips level with each other to help counter balance your muscle length differences. This isolates the legs more and keeps the lumbar spine balanced.

*Tip: Do not force these stretches or your lumbar spine and pelvis will bend and tilt out of neutral position. Contract your abdominals as you stretch. Maintain neutral posture.*

## Calf Stretch

When your calves are too tight, then your gait will be off. You will be off balance when you move and your hip and lower back will not be able to maintain correct posture. Stretching the calves will address this problem and will also be an important stretch regardless of back pain. There are numerous ways to stretch your calves. This is only one method; it helps to follow other calf stretches as well.

Step 1:  While standing upright, place both feet on the step of a staircase or block. Rest only the balls of your feet on the step. Hold on to the handrail for support and balance.

Step 2:  Relax into this stretch and wait for 1-2 minutes.

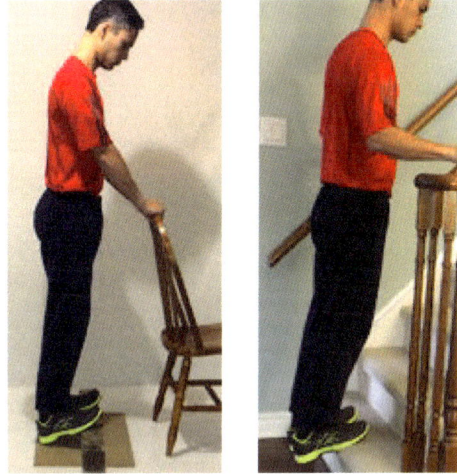

Calf muscles can tighten dramatically over time and contribute to your lower back pain indirectly through your posture and gait.

*Tip:  You can improve this stretch by performing it one foot at a time.  Footwear may be more comfortable and provide more traction.  Do not bounce or contract while performing this exercise. Flexing your toes upward will help to antagonize the calf muscles and make the stretch easier.*

## Hangs and Pushes

This exercise is simply intended to help you relieve any tension in your lower back. Depending on your weight or upper body strength and endurance, you may or may not be able to perform this exercise. If you find it too difficult or tiring, then don't place too much emphasis on them. This exercise calls for a very sturdy support. Do NOT perform them unless one is available.

## Hangs

Step 1: Using a sturdy horizontal bar, support, or pair of stable chairs, grip the supports so as to lift your upper body weight up off your lower body.

Step 2: Place your legs in front of your body so that your feet are in front and knees are bent.

Step 3: Hold for as long as is comfortable.

This is more of an endurance and strength exercise for your upper body than a rest for your lower. It is a difficult one to master because it is hard to relax the tight muscles in your lower back while contracting the upper body. This takes a lot of time, patience and strength. When you can hold this position for a long time, you will be able to feel the muscles of the lower spine relax to relieve some of your lower back pain.

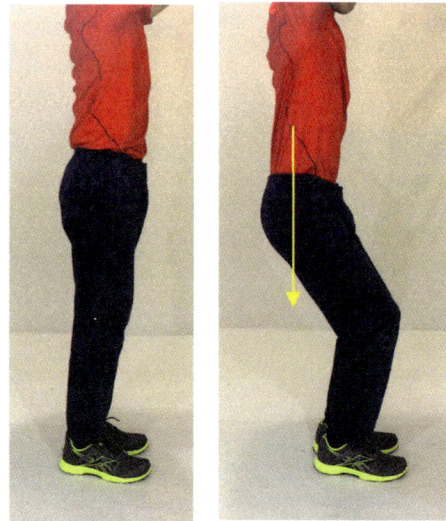

*Tip: Do not let your pelvis tilt forward while hanging as it will only increase pressure on the lumbar discs. Keep your knees out in front and maintain a neutral posture.*

## Pushes

In order to do this exercise, you will need to wear a pant or short that has a belt inserted.

Step 1: While lying down on the floor face up, bring your feet closer to your buttocks to bend the knees and hips. Keep the knees up and together.

Step 2: Place both hands beside you and grip your belt on both sides. Push down to elongate your spine evenly and hold for as long as possible.

Step 3: Rest and push intermittently.

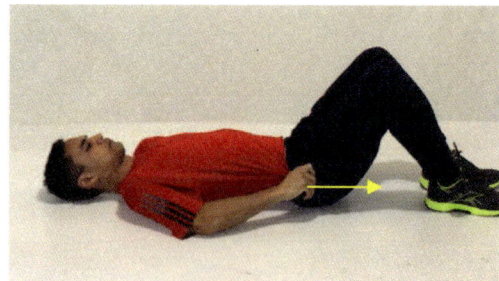

Application: While lying down in bed or on the couch. Usually before bed.

## Lying Twist

The lying twist is similar to many other exercises that are practiced to help with low back pain. When you perform this stretch, your upper back muscles will relax and stretch before your lower back muscles will. This one allows you to use gravity to relax into the stretch. By crossing your legs, you can increase the mobility in your hips. Holding your hands together and lowering one elbow to the side will help to keep your back flat to the floor as your legs rotate. Take time to hold this stretch to allow the lower back muscles to finally release and elongate.

Step 1:  Lie back on the floor with your knees bent and feet on the floor. Hold your hands together.

Step 2:  Cross your legs and slowly relax over to the side. The leg on top should lean both legs to its own side. Place your elbow on the opposite side for support to keep the back on the floor.

Step 3:  Relax. Hold this position for 30 seconds to 2 minutes.

Step 4:  Repeat with the other side.

Step 5:  Repeat often.

This exercise will stretch very tight and resistant muscles. You may feel sore afterwards as tight and weak muscles will be stretched. Allow time to recover. This stretch requires time to become effective as the lowest muscles on the spine are difficult to mobilize from over tightness.

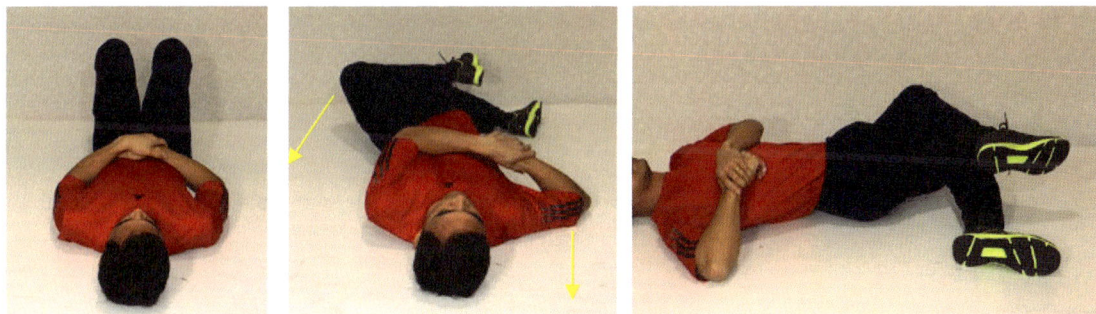

*Tip: Let gravity do the work. To strengthen the muscles stretched, slowly bring them back up folded to the original position without assistance.*

## Abdominal Crunch

Abdominal crunches are very popular but can performed in many ways. Some ways are more effective than others. This variation is done to help condition the abdominals so as to protect the lumbar vertebrae from excessive arching.

Step 1: Lie comfortably on your back on a padded floor. Raise your knees and feet up together to elevate them off of the floor.

Step 2: Raise your arms out in front pointing them straight at your toes, almost touching your knees.

Step 3: Contract your abdominals that are near your belly button and slowly bring your hands closer to your feet.

Step 4: Pause for 5-10 seconds while breathing. Press the small of your back into the floor and gently lift the edge of your buttocks off of the floor.

Step 5: Relax back down to the floor.

Step 6: Repeat this exercise for as long as you can to improve your muscular strength and endurance.

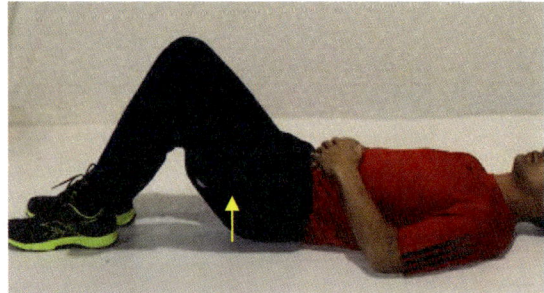

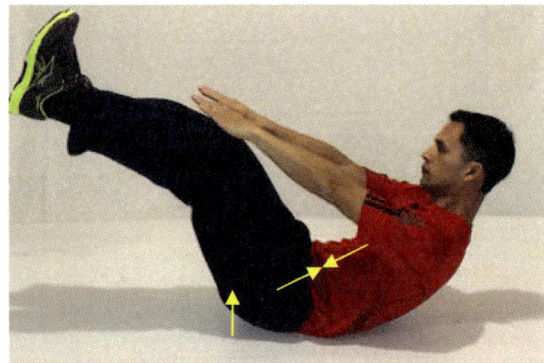

*Tip: Avoid leaning your head forward and overexerting your neck muscles. Your neck muscles may be the first to fatigue in this exercise. Rest them often to protect them. If you can place your hands above the knees, it will help to balance your hold.*

*Application: After waking and prior to bedtime.*

## Quadriceps Stretch

Tight quadriceps can exacerbate lower back pain.  They cause your pelvis to tilt forward.  The lower discs bulge and the facet joints bear too much pressure.  This stretch will lengthen the rectus femoris and allow the pelvis to tilt backward to a more neutral angle.  Combine this stretch with abdominal exercises.   This exercise is the same as the previous hamstring stretch but it is done without support and trains you to balance fully on one leg.

Step 1: Stand upright with a neutral posture and abdominals gently contracted.

Step 2:  Grasp one leg at the ankle and raise it from behind close to your buttock.  Keep your hips level and maintain a gentle abdominal contraction.

Step 3:  Hold for 30 seconds to 2 minutes.  Rest back down.

Step 4:  Repeat with the other leg.

Step 5:  Repeat often.

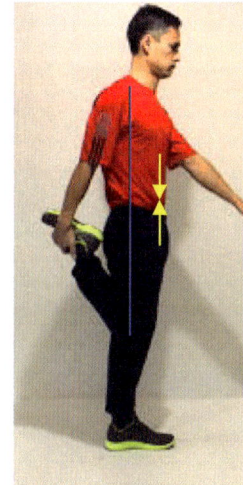

As your quadriceps lengthen,  your pelvic tilt will become more neutral.  Try to contract your abdominals as you perform this stretch to counter the forward tilt that the stretch creates while it is tight.  Avoid pulling too hard on your ankle to prevent unnecessary injury to your knee.

*Tip:  As your quads lengthen, you can improve and lengthen the stretch:*
*Support the stretched leg by moving it further behind you on an armrest of your couch,*
*while holding your ankle.*

*Application: Anytime that you are standing.*

## Seated Knee Raise

This exercise helps initiate muscular strength in the hips and abdominals. It is important to perform them unassisted and often. At first, your mobility and strength may be limited but try to bring the knee up high to your chest and try to pause. Strong hip flexors and abdominals will help prevent excessive anterior pelvic tilt. It will also give strength to your gluteus muscles.

Step 1: Sit upright in a comfortable seat. Put your hands on your legs or on the side of the seat. Lean forward slightly and contract the abdominals gently.

Step 2: Raise one knee up as high as you can and hold. Keep your buttocks firmly seated on the chair. Avoid raising one up as you lift the knee.

Step 3: Rest back down.

Step 4: Repeat with the other leg and alternate sides often.

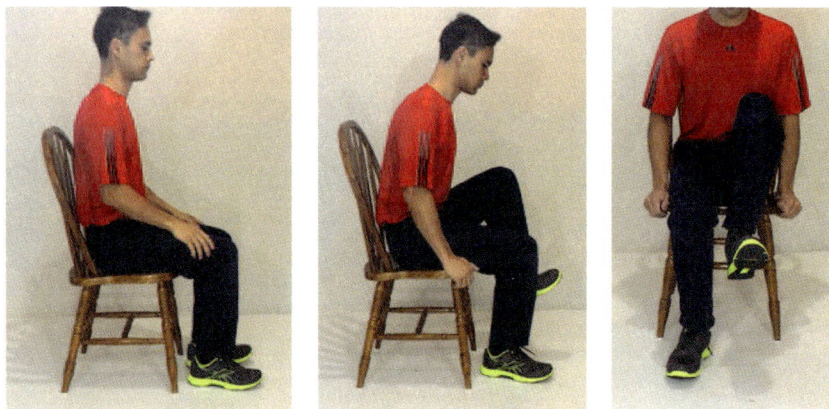

*Tip: Keep your lower back perpendicular to the seat and focus on keeping both of your sit bones firmly on the seat. Time and relaxation will help facilitate this.*

*Application: Prior to rising from bed. Dressing with your socks and shoes while seated.*

## Progressive Exercises

### Seated Hip Adjustment (assisted)

This exercise gets the hips and pelvis mobile and loosens the tight muscles involved. You may find it uncomfortable at first because it is meant to move a very weak and tight area that will be very resistant. This movement will be performed again in the Challenge Exercises, but with more muscular exertion. For now, you will only need gravity to help you with the adjustments. You will need a soft cover book or any flat object to assist you. (0.5 to 1.5 inch thickness preferred.)

Step 1:  Sit upright on a comfortable but firm seat.

Step 2:  Place the flat object under one buttock, beginning with a 0.5 inch thickness.

Step 3:  Relax into the object while keeping your spine vertical. Hold for at least 2 minutes.

Step 4:  Repeat on other side.

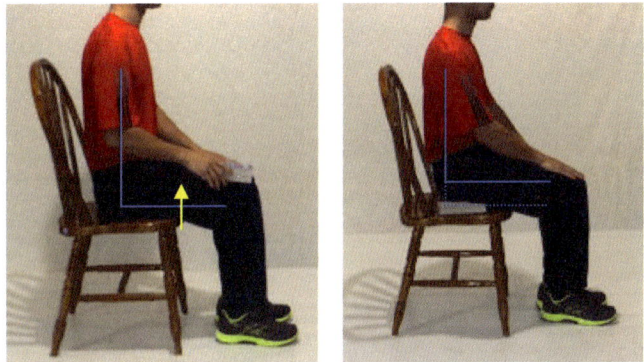

You may not feel any movement or adjustments at first due to tightness. It will take time. As you slowly start to move with gravity, maintain an upright posture. The adjustment may start to feel uncomfortable as muscles are being stretched and moved after a long period of immobility. This exercise may make you feel sore afterwards. Rest often. In time, the exercise will become easier to perform with little discomfort.

*Tip: If you find it easy and your posture remains upright, then increase the thickness of the flat object anywhere up to 2 inches.*

## Seated and Floor Hip Shift

This exercise is similar to the previous one in that it targets hip and pelvis stiffness. This time you will need to use your hip and leg muscles to generate the shifts. It is a very easy exercise but may be uncomfortable due to tightness. You may feel that you cannot actually perform this exercise, but with increased strength and time, you will progress and feel less discomfort. The more that you shift, the more you are calling tight and weak muscles into action. They will feel tired and sore afterwards. Rest often.

The floor version of the hip shift is slightly easier but both are recommended.

### Seated Version

Step 1: Use any seat available. Keeping your legs parallel together, gently slide one leg forward and the other backward. Use your hands to elevate you for support if needed. Stay upright and keep your stomach pointing forward.

Step 2: Slide as much as possible comfortably. Hold for a count of 5-10 seconds.

Step 3: Slide and return back to your original seated position.

Step 4: Repeat with the other leg forward and backward instead.

Step 5: Repeat both sides again as long as you are able.

It is important to keep the lumbar spine facing forward as this exercise is meant to move the hips and not the spine.
*Tip: Pushing up on the seat with your hands will help to take pressure off of the spine. To make this shift more effective, slightly rotate or twist your body towards the leg that is moving forward and hold.*

Step 6: Using your hands, push down on the seat to lighten your body weight. Elevate one thigh and buttock slowly off the seat while pushing down with the other thigh and buttock.

Step 7: Hold for 5-10 seconds. Relax back down.

Step 8: Repeat with other side.

Step 9: Repeat entire exercise (from step 6) with other side.

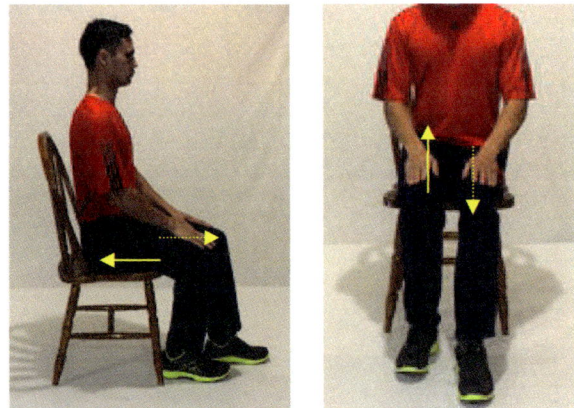

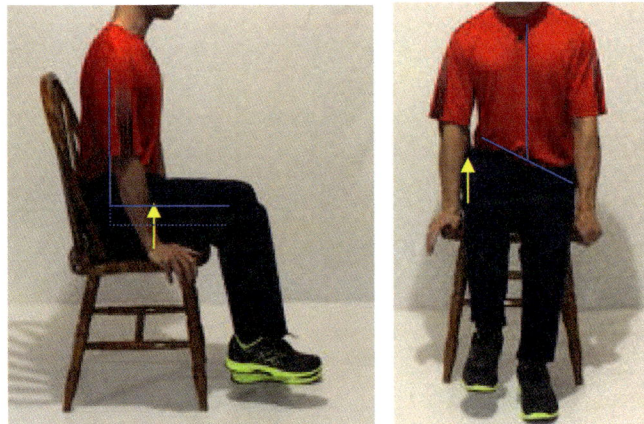

Remember to keep your spine vertical during this exercise. This exercise helps to loosen tight lumbar muscles and to improve your balance.

Floor Version

Step 1:  Place both hands and knees on the floor and looking toward the floor.  Your arms and legs should be perpendicular to the floor.  Elevate one thigh vertically off the ground as far as is comfortable. Keep both of your thighs parallel to one another.

Step 2:  Hold for 5-10 seconds.  Relax back down.

Step 3:  Repeat with the other leg.

Step 4:  Repeat entire exercise with both sides often to increase your mobility.

Step 5:  Return back to original position.  Position one knee slightly forward/further ahead on the floor (knee A) and the other slightly down/further away on the floor (knee B).  Keep both of your thighs perpendicular to the floor.

Step 6:  Without moving your hands and knees, flex the hip of the forward leg forward and extend the hip of the downward leg backward.  Use your hip muscles to rotate the pelvis while keeping the spine straight.  Keep both of your thighs perpendicular to the floor.

Step 7:  Hold for 5-10 seconds. Relax.

Step 8:  Repeat with the other side.

Step 9: Repeat entire exercise (from step 5) often.

*Tip:  This is a static contraction exercise.  Try to keep your spine straight as you flex your hip muscles. Keep your thighs parallel to each other and perpendicular to the floor.*

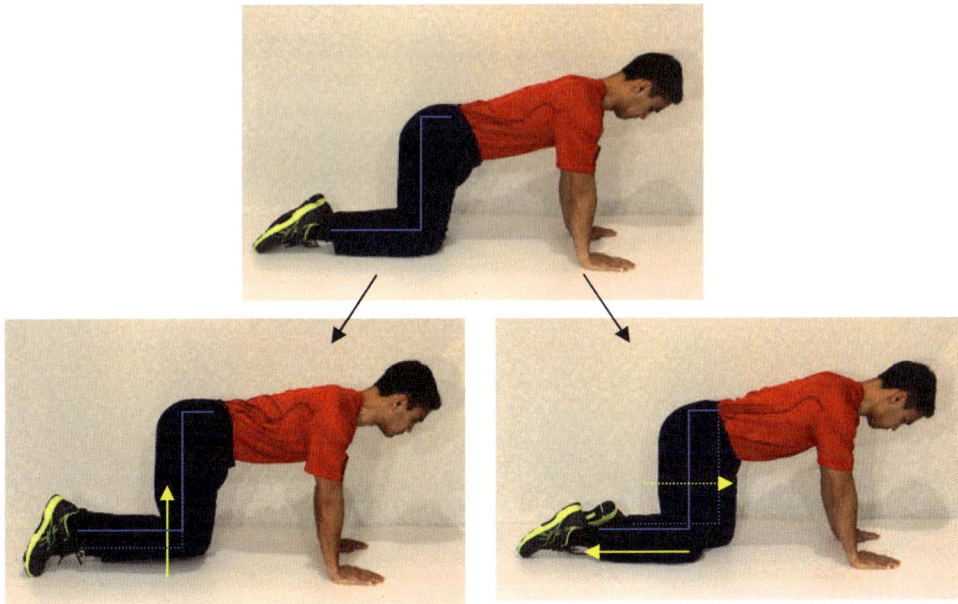

## Seated Leg Rotation (assisted with contraction)

This exercise will help you to improve the rotational ability of your femur. When your femur does not rotate well, it will affect the tilt of your pelvis and subsequently your posture and lumbar curve. Some people may already rotate very well in one direction but poorly in the other (anterior vs. posterior). Try to perform this exercise often enough to be balanced.

Step 1: While seated, elevate one leg slightly off the floor. Rotate it outward to the side as far as possible and hold for 5 seconds. Lean forward slightly and use your hand to assist in rotating the leg further.

Step 2: Rotate the same leg inward and past the other leg to the opposite side and hold for 5 seconds. Return and relax.

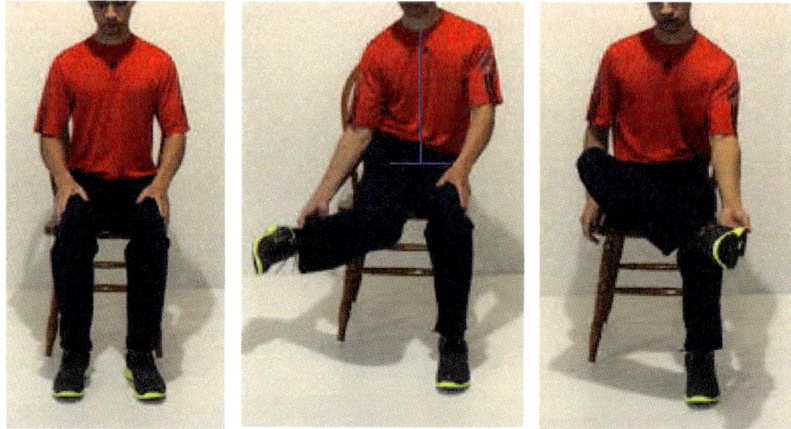

Step 3: Repeat with the other leg.

Step 4: Repeat the entire exercise often.

There may not be very much movement in one direction at first compared to the other. External rotation is generally harder. You may feel minimal gains at first if your muscles are tight and weak. If you have any knee issues, be very careful not to place excess stress on your knee when rotating your leg.

*Tip: Use your hands to assist you or hold on to your pant leg if needed.*

## Seated Leg Cross with forward lean

This is a stationary exercise and is meant to both mobilize and open the hips, and stretch the leg and hip muscles. You will mobilize the hip joint while keeping the pelvis and lumbar spine straight. You want to minimize bending of the back and to allow the hip joint to control the forward lean instead.

Step 1: Sit on the floor and maintain an upright posture. Cross your legs.

Step 2: Slowly lean forward but begin at the area below the belly button. Lean forward as though you are trying to press this area into your ankles in front of you. Only move as far as you can while maintaining this posture.

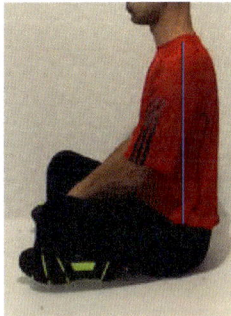

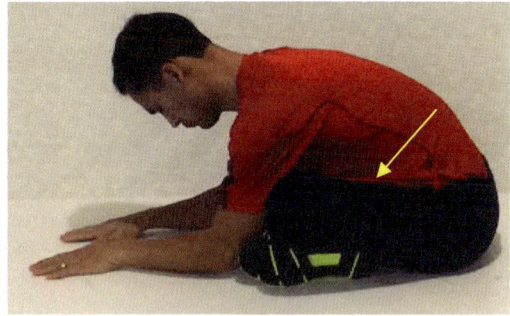

Step 3: Hold for 1-2 minutes while using your hands to support your forward lean.

At first, there may not be very much forward lean. You may find yourself bending at the lower back. Do not do this. You want to bend only at the hip joint. The back must remain straight. Go only as far as your knees will allow to protect your knee joint.

*Tip: You can vary this exercise, by placing one folded leg fully overlaid on the other folded leg and by alternating sides between each hold. Relax into this forward lean.*

## Floor Leg Bend and Shift

This exercise encourages your hip mobility and helps you to keep your posture. When you are able to perform this well, you will find it easier and more comfortable to sit on the floor or a chair without back support. You will need your hands to assists you at first. Eventually you will be able to perform the movement hands free and more quickly.

Step 1: Sit on the floor with your legs crossed and posture straight and upright.

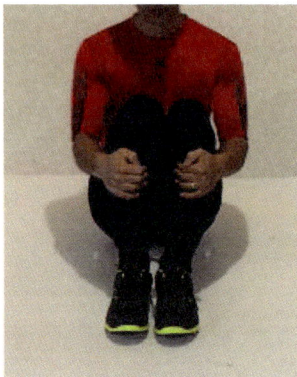

Step 2: Move one leg out slightly to the side while maintaining the bend.

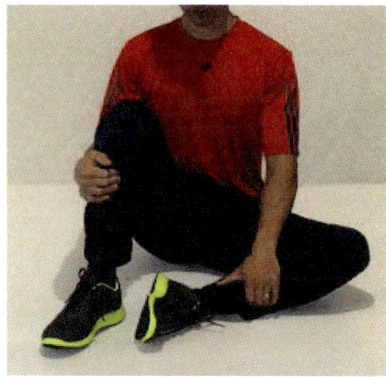

Step 3: Using your hands, slowly slide the other leg out and straighten it out in front of you. Keep your posture upright.

Step 4: Slowly pull the same leg out and to the same side while bending at the knee. Try to rest the inside of the shin on the floor. Move only as far as is comfortable.

Step 5: Hold for at least 30 seconds to as long as you feel comfortable.

Step 6: Repeat with the other side.

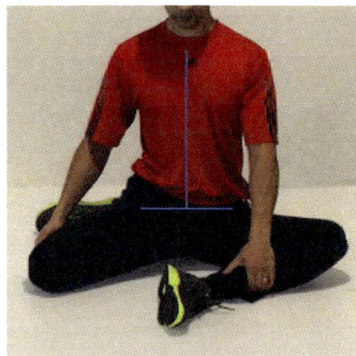

When you hold this exercise, one side of your buttocks will tend to naturally lift off of the floor. Depending on your flexibility, it will gradually settle closer to the floor. Not everyone can do this. Do not force this stretch.

Try to avoid leaning and keep upright. This is difficult at first but is preferred. As in the previous exercise, use caution with your knee joint.

*Tip: If you find this exercise too difficult to perform at first, you can elevate your seat higher off the ground with a cushion and work your way lower later on.*

*You can get more out of this exercise by: a) switching your legs back and forth from one side to the other, b) repeating this movement, c) performing it without the assistance of your hands, and d) at a faster pace. This is easier to do once your hip mobility has improved.*

## Seated Leg to Chest

This is a static stretch exercise meant to target the muscles of the buttocks (gluteus). When they are too tight, your hips will not flex well and your back will bend to compensate. This exercise requires extensive amounts of time in order for them to resist stretching and relax. Do not rush through this exercise.

Step 1: While seated, raise one knee up and bring the inner thigh up toward your chest. Use your hands to carefully assist in rotating the leg inward to your chest.

Step 2: Hold for 2 minutes while keeping your back straight.

Step 3: Relax back down and repeat with the other leg.

Step 4: Repeat often.

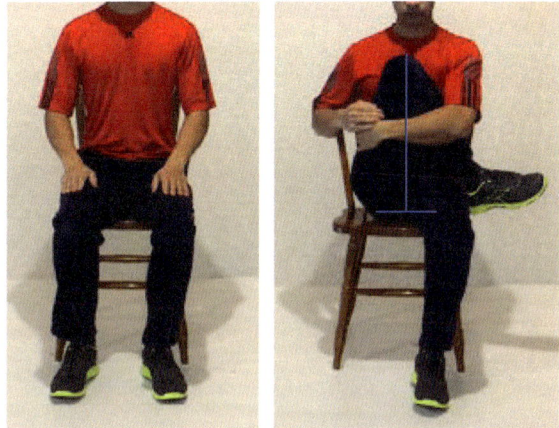

It may take time before you can bring your inner thigh to your chest. Make sure that your lower back does not bend during this hold. You should feel a very strong pull in the buttocks area as well as near the outside above the knee joint. The pull will change in sensation as the muscle learns to relax and stretch.

Be careful not to pull on your ankle to assist with the internal rotation when bringing your inner thigh up. This can place unnecessary stress on the knee joint.

*Application: Watching TV*

## Leaning Hip Shift

This is the same exercise as the previous hip shifts but requires you to stand and lean over with assistance. You will find this easy to perform when you are engaged with any activity that uses the same position (ex. using the bathroom sink).  This exercise is more advanced than the previous hip shift because it helps to stretch your hamstrings.

Step 1:  Stand in front of a counter or chair with feet shoulder width apart.  Lean over the counter while using your arms or elbows for support and height.  Keep your pelvis and lower back in line with each other and straight.

Step 2: While keeping both feet on the same spot on the ground, bend one knee and straighten the other. Move and flex the forward knee closer to the counter or chair, while straightening the rear leg.

Step 3: Contract both legs and hold for 1-2 seconds.

Step 4: Quickly alternate with the other side is the same fashion.

Step 5: Rock back and forth for about 1-2 minutes.

This exercise is great for stretching the hamstrings and mobilizing your hips.

*Tip:  Flex your hip muscles vigorously to stimulate mobility.*

*Application:  When using your sink to brush your teeth or wash your face.*

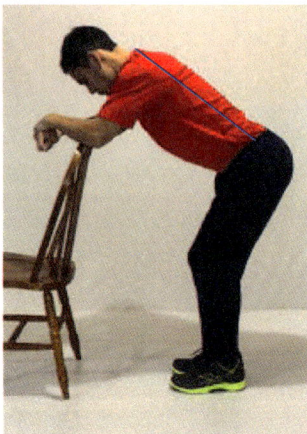

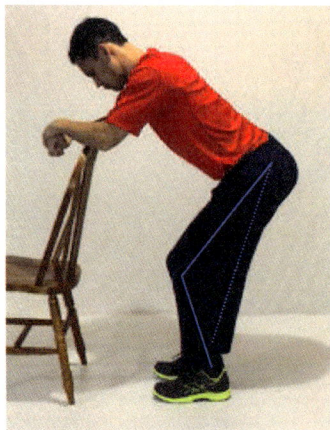

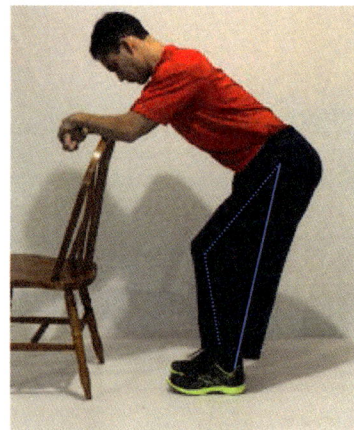

## Rail Squat (assisted)

At this time it is important develop your leg muscles.  The primary mover of your legs should be your gluteus muscles.  They must activate and function first in order to give you the power and movement for your legs.  This helps to relieve stress on the lower back.  This exercise will help you regain this function.

Step 1:  Stand in front of a rail or banister grasping the rail with your hands.  Place your feet together and bring your toes close to the bottom of the rail.

Step 2:  While keeping your arms straight, slowly lower your body to the ground until your thighs are horizontal to the floor.

Step 3: Hold this position for 2 seconds and *slowly* raise back up.

Step 4: Repeat this exercise 5-10 times.

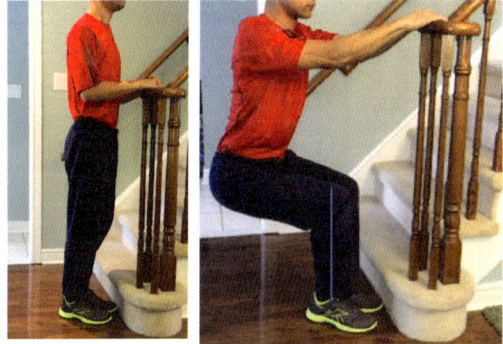

As you lower your body, keep your arms straight, and your shins vertical.  If you cannot lower yourself to horizontal (half squat) then only lower to a quarter squat and then progress to a half when possible.

*Tip:  You can vary this exercise in many ways to improve your leg strength further.  Variations include: widening your foot stance,  lowering your squat height further; also straightening one leg out to the side and bearing most of the weight on the bent leg.   You can rest one outside ankle (resting leg) over on to the knee of the other (active leg) to increase a gluteus stretch of the resting leg.*

## Seated Hamstring Stretch

This is one of the most important exercises in this program. Tight hamstrings have a large impact on chronic back pain. They prevent your pelvis from tilting forward with your spine as you lean forward. Your spine should have a stable, neutral curve as you lean forward and the pelvis must tilt with it to protect the lower discs. If your spine bends in this region, the lower back muscles that support it will overstretch, become fatigued and very sore, adding to your pain. The wrong muscles may compensate and result in a back spasm.

Unfortunately, most of the stretches for hamstrings out there do more harm than good to your lower back. Do not lean forward to bend over to touch your toes in order to stretch your hamstrings. You will injure your back because your pelvis is not tilted with your spine. You are simply bending at your spine which is harmful.

It is important to master the deep squat rest in order to benefit from this stretch.

*Practice this stretch often and try to stretch your hamstrings as often as possible.*

Step 1: Sit down on a soft carpet for comfort. Keep your back straight and bring your knees to your chest. Hold them with your arms and bring your belly button area firmly against your thighs. Do not move to step 2 unless you are firmly and comfortably maintaining contact between your belly and thighs. Squeeze gently as though you are trying to hold a flat piece of paper in between.

Step 2: Hold your feet firmly with both hands. Make sure that you feel that your pelvis and lumbar spine are aligned and engaged with your thighs. Slowly extend your legs out but *keep* your belly against your thighs. This will preserve your lumbar and pelvic curve together. Maintain a grip on your feet.

Step 3: Extend your legs slowly inch by inch and as far and as comfortably as you can. Hold for 1-2 minutes.

Step 4: Rest and repeat.

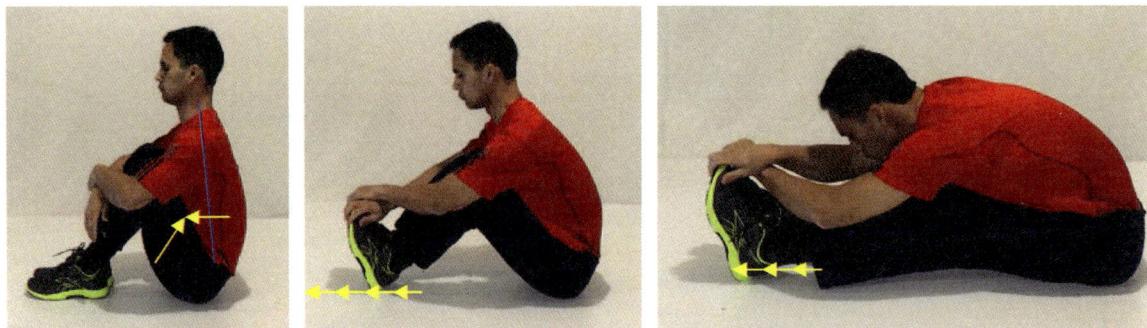

The only part of your body that is moving during this exercise should be your lower legs as they extend out in front of you. You can shuffle your feet forward as tension in the hamstrings fades. This is not an easy or even pleasant stretch at first because your hamstrings, pelvis and lower back muscles are unbalanced at this point. This exercise attempts to bring back this balance and to help to realign the femur with the pelvis. You may not extend well in the beginning but if you persist, you will progress. As you progress in the program, there will be a more advanced form of this stretch.

## Stair Step (up and down)

This exercise is straight forward.  Please use the handrails for assistance.  Keep both your back and forward shin vertical and avoid leaning them forward.  The goal is to exercise and strengthen the gluteus muscles and not the quads.  Start with one step only at first,  when this becomes too easy,  move up to two steps.  Three steps is a challenge but provides maximum muscle activation. When you step back down, keep your shin and back in vertical position and use the handrails for balance.

Step 1:  Stand in front of a staircase and hold on to the handrails.

Step 2:  Place one foot on the step and position it until the shin is vertical.

Step 3:  Keep your back straight and step up slowly.  Take approximately 1-2 seconds to complete the movement. Use the handrails to maintain your position and balance. Rest on the upper step.

Step 4: Slowly step back down to the original standing position.  Maintain shin and back position and use the rails.  Take 1-2 seconds to compete the movement. Rest on lower step.

Step 5:  Repeat with the other leg.

Step 6: Repeat entire exercise often.

*Tip:  Contract the glutes and not the quads.*

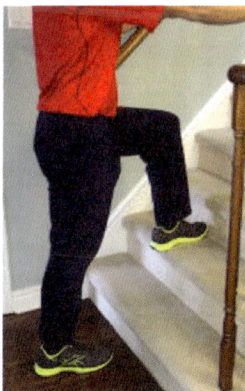

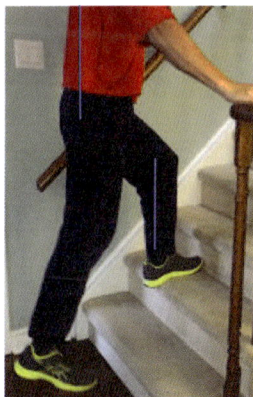

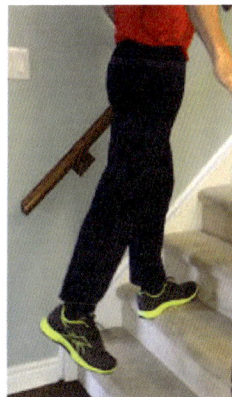

## Reverse Stair Squat Lean

You will be targeting and mobilizing your hips in this exercise one side at a time. The stairs are an effective way to enhance this stretch.

Step 1: Stand on a stair looking down while holding onto the rails. Lean forward to ensure that your back is straight and pelvis is tilted forward with it.

Step 2: Lift one foot up and behind you. Try to keep this foot flat on the step.

Step 3: Slowly lean forward more while shifting your buttocks backward and out to the side (about 45 degrees). Try to straighten the lower leg

Step 4: Hold for 1-5 seconds.

Step 5: Repeat both sides.

*Avoid leaning your upper shin forward excessively. This will help to prevent stress to the knee joint.*

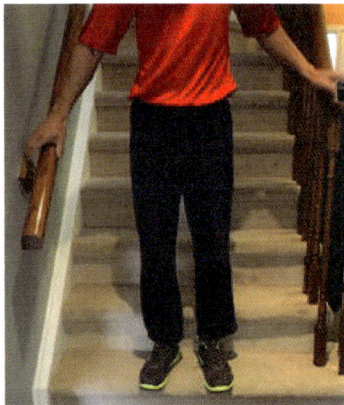

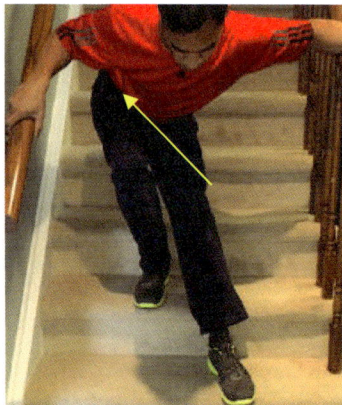

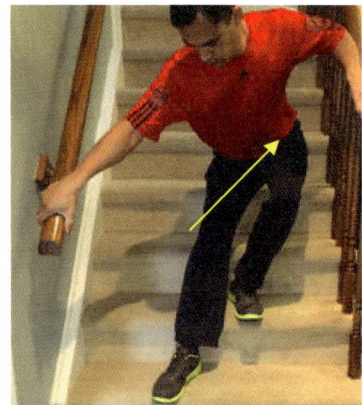

## Hip Opener (inside and outside)

This is similar to the deep squat rest and the seated hamstring stretch but uses the thigh muscles more. This exercise will help to loosen you up more and strengthen your leg muscles.

Step 1: Sit in the deep squat rest position. Grab both ankles from the front. Keep your belly against your thighs. Position your arms on the outside of your legs.

Step 2: Lift your buttocks up sufficiently until you can get your elbows inside of your legs. Then lower yourself back down.

Step 3: Repeat until you have moved your elbows to the outside of your legs again.

Step 4: Repeat this exercise often.

*Tip: You can improve this exercise by widening your foot stance and by raising and lowering yourself slowly.*

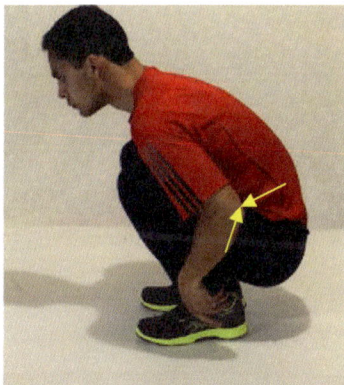

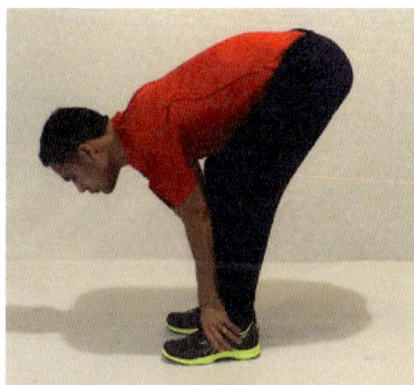

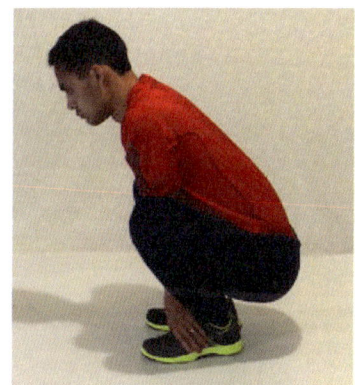

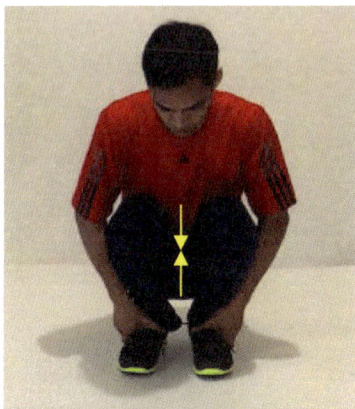

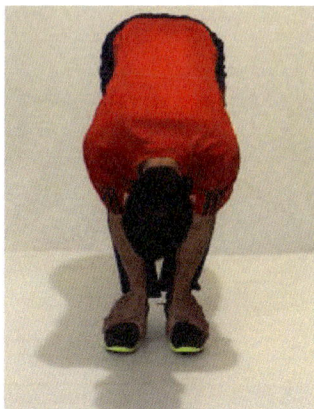

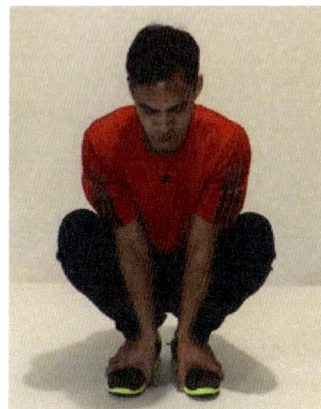

## Seated Calf Stretch

Calf muscles are stubborn and always require constant attention because they are used everyday. If they are tight, they will affect your lower back via your stride, stance and your posture. This exercise will also help to stretch the hamstrings.

Step 1: Sit on a chair. Raise one leg up to your chest while holding it up with your hands.

Step 2: Flex your toes toward you. Hold your feet with your hands. Elevate your leg and extend it out as far as possible.

Step 3: You can either choose to hold this stretch, or immediately return back to your chest.

Step 4: Repeat with the other leg.

Step 5: Repeat entire exercise often.

When you extend your leg, do not apply too much force as you do not want to strain your back. You want to use the arms to help elevate the leg but with minimal help.

*Tip: Keep the toes flexed toward you. The higher the elevation, the more effective the stretch. Allow your hip flexors to elevate the leg more than with your arms.*

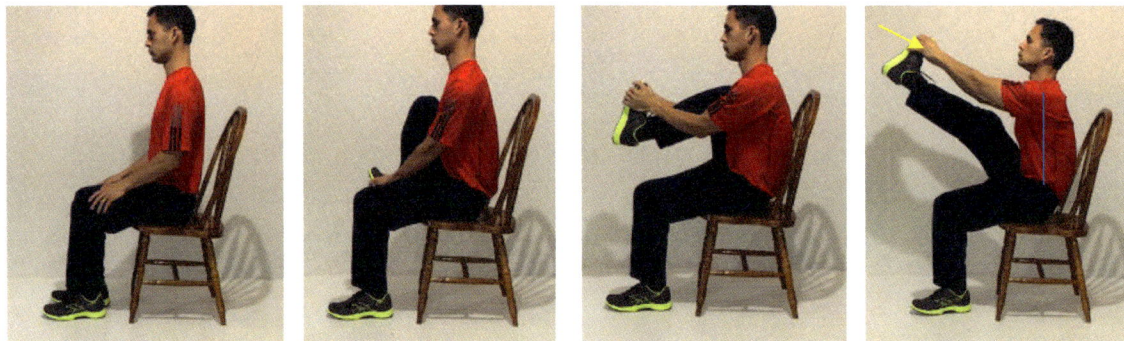

## Double Leg Rotation

This is the same exercise as in the previous seated leg rotations but this time without the assistance. With this exercise, you can gain significant mobility in your hip joint. This exercise requires bent leg movement. It is important to use only your leg muscles without using your hands to develop strength.

Step 1: Sit on the edge of a seat with your back upright and knees apart slightly.

Step 2: Elevate one leg and rotate the leg out in one direction as far as possible. Pause for 1 second. Rest and bring down.

Step 3: Elevate the same leg and rotate the leg out in the opposite direction as far as possible. Pause for 1 second. Rest and bring down.

Step 4: Repeat with the other leg.

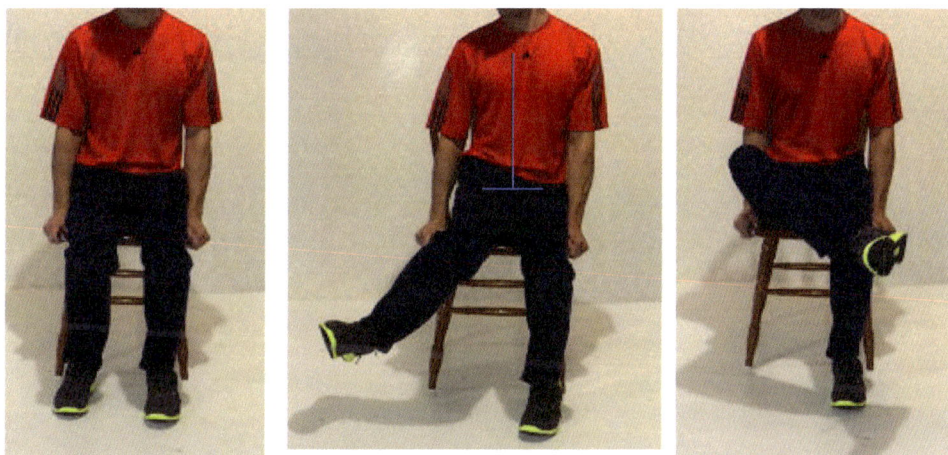

Step 5: Repeat this entire exercises, but while standing upright.

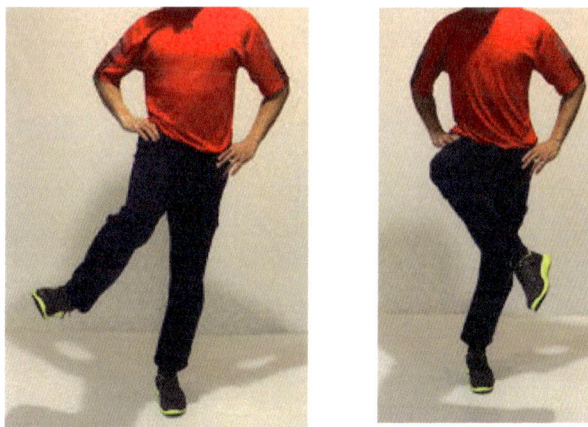

You may not be able to rotate your leg in one direction as well the other. This reflects your tightness and muscle imbalance. Also, it is normal for there to be a difference but when it is too unbalanced, it can lead to pelvic tilt issues and back pain.

## Deep Abdominal Crunch (leg raised)

Abdominal crunches are common and effective. Perform these often. Avoid straining your neck and upper body. You need to be familiar with the small of the back. It is the slight space in behind the lumbar curve which provides a slight forward curve. If it is too exaggerated, it will contribute to excessive curve, anterior pelvic tilt, and back pain. When you are fully lying on the ground with your legs straight, this curve should be very slight. Only enough to squeeze your flat hand in between. The more success you have in creating a flat small of your back, the more relief you will have.

Step 1: Lying back on the floor, locate the small of the back. Elevate your legs slightly and keep them together.

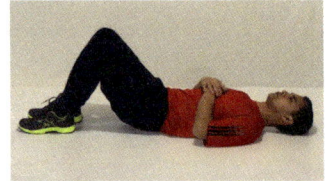

Step 2: Cross your arms and raise your chest toward your knees.

Step 3: Contract the abdominal muscles that are on the opposite side of the small of your back and lower to your groin. Tilt your pelvis up towards you. Hold for 10 seconds. Return to rest position.

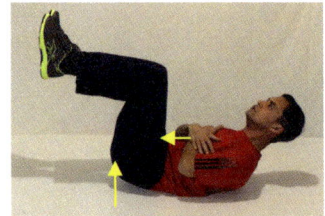

Step 4: Repeat often.

It is not the six-pack that you are targeting but the lowest abdominal muscle involved. This exercise requires a posterior pelvic tilt at the same time to enhance contraction of the lower abdominals.

*Tip: Tilt as though you were trying elevate your tail bone to place a small book underneath. Focus on contracting your lower abdominals rather than your upper.*

*Application: After waking and prior to bed.*

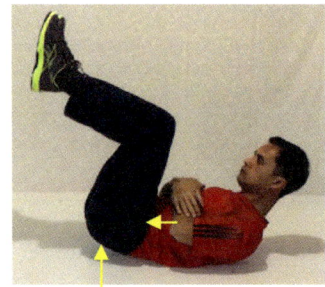

## Plank with Steps

The plank will help to strengthen your core and virtually all of your muscles from head to toe. You want to keep your entire body straight without slumping to the floor. Slumping will contribute to back pain. Adding leg steps are intended to improve abdominal strength and hip mobility.

Step 1: Lie forward in a push up position. Toes on the ground feet together. Hands on the ground, arms straight and shoulder width apart.

Step 2: While keeping your back straight, raise one knee up toward your chest and pause for 1 second. Return, to original position.

Step 3: Repeat with the other leg.

Step 4: Repeat the entire exercise often.

You can raise the difficulty of this exercise by holding your knee forward for longer periods of time or by performing the plank on your elbows. You will need to bend at the hips slightly to adjust for the leg step.

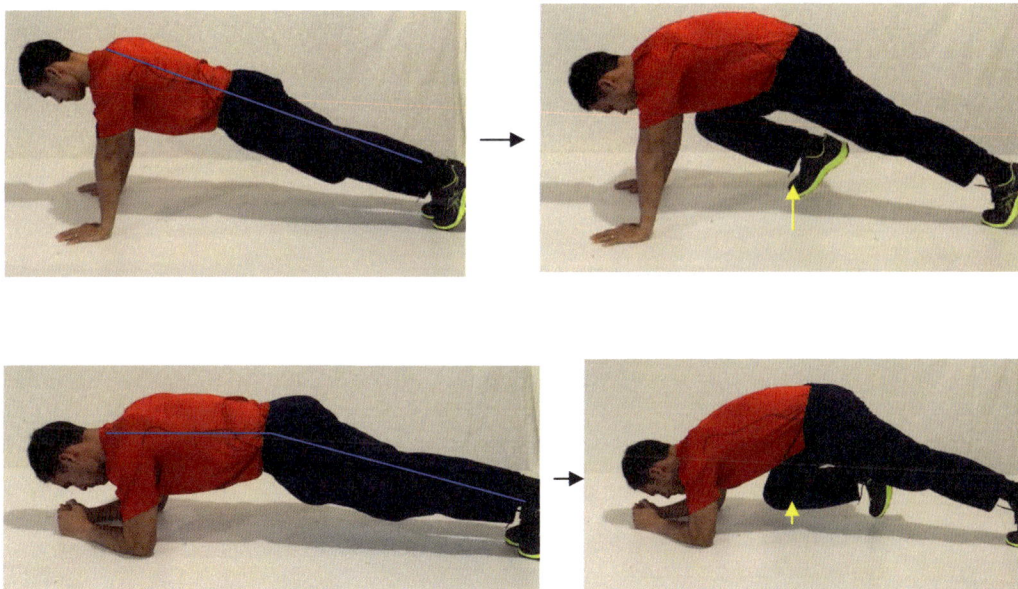

## Couch Split

Couch splits are simply that. Splits on the couch. As you move into the splits, use your upper body to support and balance yourself. Do not force this stretch. Ease into it slowly. You can position your forward leg off the side of the couch for assistance. Slide your rear leg backward to increase your stretch. Use the flexion and contraction of your leg muscles to facilitate the stretch and rely less on gravity to lower yourself down.

Step 1: Start in a gentle split position with your forward foot on the ground. Hold on to the couch for support and balance if needed. Keep your pelvis pointed forward and stay upright.

Step 2: Slide your rear leg backward slowly and pause for 1 minute. Return to a rest position. Keep your rear leg in a parallel line with your forward leg.

Step 3: Repeat the other side

Step 4: Repeat the other side often.

When you perform this stretch, your pelvis may rotate out to the side. By keeping the pelvis forward, you will have a more effective stretch. To *fully* lower the pelvis, the hip will eventually need to tilt out to the side. Be careful not to strain the rear knee when you hold it.

*Tip: To improve this stretch, slide backward until you can elevate the forward leg off of the ground. It is important to keep the pelvis faced forward initially.*

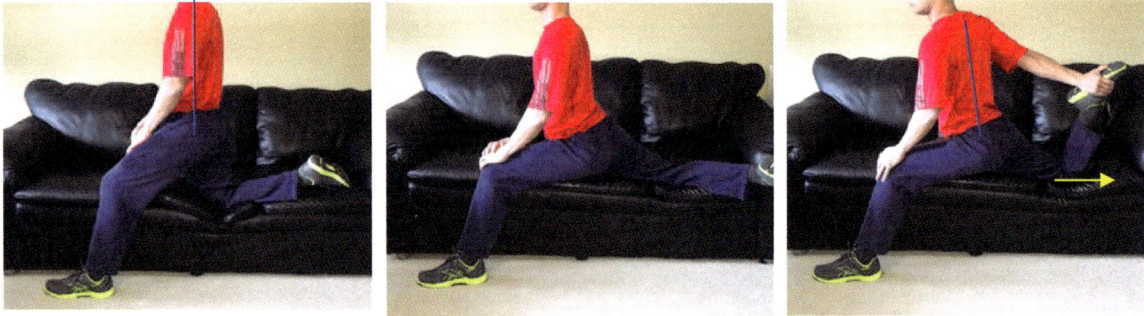

## Outside Hip Stretch

This exercise is very challenging but is considered progressive because it takes significant time to accomplish. Allow your body weight to help you to ease in to the final stretch position. Make sure that you use your abdominals to bring your belly to the floor and avoid bending over. This exercise may place pressure on the knee joint. Use caution and ease in to the stretch only as far as your knees will allow.

Step 1: Place your hands and knees on the floor. Slowly cross your legs from behind and bring one knee behind the other. Feet should now be on opposite sides with outside shins resting on the floor. Keep your hands on the floor out in front of you.

Step 2: Slowly ease back and sit carefully down. Maintain leaning forward with a strong abdominal contraction. Actively bring your belly toward your legs. Try to keep your hands on the floor in front of you.

Step 3: Hold for 30 second to 2 minutes. Relax and rest.

Step 4: Repeat with alternate legs crossed.

Step 4: Repeat often as long your knees and lower back are comfortable.

If you find this to be too challenging, then simply ease to your own limit and hold at that point. When your stretch improves, you will be able to move back further with your legs at a more pronounced angle. Try to keep the knees close to each other if possible. If you cannot do this, then work at your preferred position.

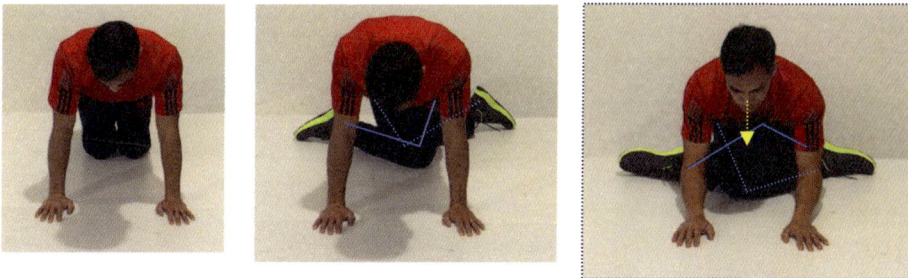

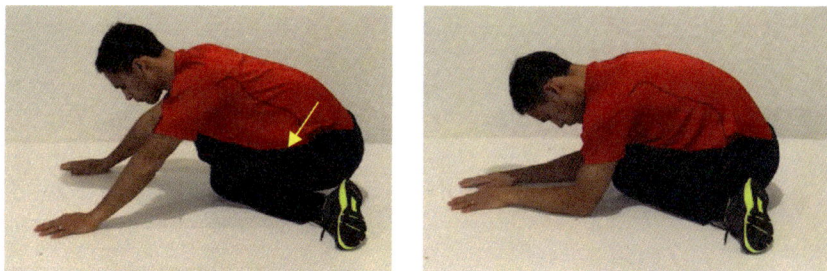

## Standing Abdominal

This exercise will help counteract forward pelvic tilt and associated back pain when standing for long periods of time. You can perform this exercise at any time that your are standing.

Step 1: Stand upright feet together. Contract the gluteus muscles.

Step 2: Contract the abdominal muscles so as to tilt your belly button up towards you while drawing your belly button in toward your spine.

Step 3: Hold for 5-10 seconds.

Step 4: Repeat often.

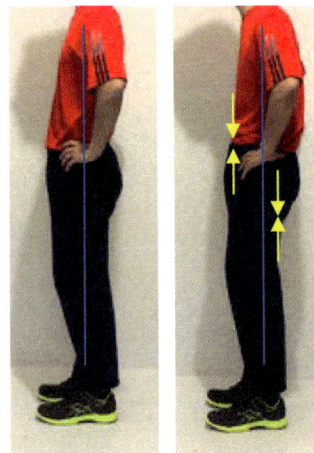

Be conscious to keep your neck relaxed, as this exercise will cause your neck to bend forward

*Tip: You can place your hands on your hips to help rock them upward in a posterior tilt. Try to increase the amount of time that you hold this exercise to improve your endurance and to help release the tightness in your quadriceps.*

# Challenging Exercises

### Seated Leg Lift (multidirectional)

This exercise requires you to use your leg muscles to elevate your leg. You will need to lift each leg in up to five different angles. Forward, forward-side, side, side- backward and backward. While performing each of these exercises, maintain both your balance and upright posture. It will help to use a chair with a backrest for support.

Step 1: Sit on a chair with the inside thigh fully on the seat and the other thigh elevated off the seat. Use the chair rest to support you and maintain an upright posture.

Step 2: Raise your elevated leg forward until straight. Pause for 1 second and return to rest position.

Step 3: Repeat but with the following angles: forward-side, side, side-backward and backward.

Step 4: Repeat with other leg.

Step 5: Repeat entire exercise as often as is comfortable.

You may not be able to fully elevate horizontally and with a straight leg but try to perform with this movement in mind.

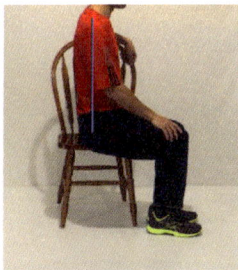

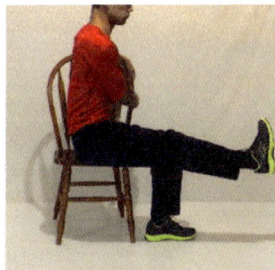

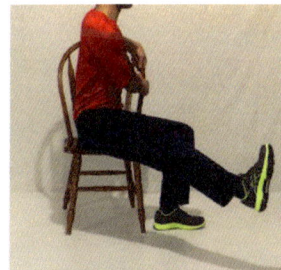

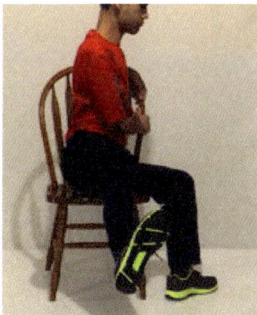

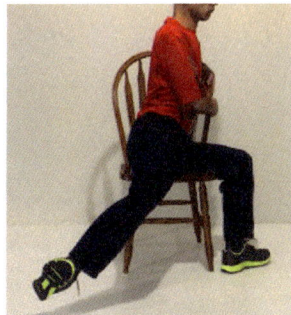

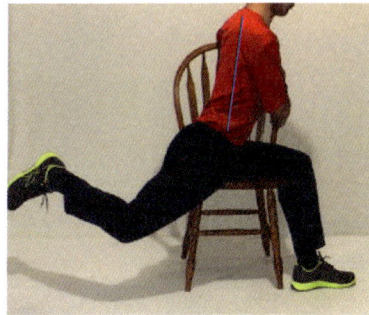

## Advanced Hamstring Stretch (ankle and floor)

This is one of the most important and fundamental stretches in the program. Do this one as often as you can so that you may be able to achieve as straight a leg position as possible. Everyone has different leg length and arm length ratios. Adjust your hand grip as needed to accommodate this difference and to preserve the effectiveness of this stretch. *You do not need to straighten your legs to fully benefit from this exercise. Stretch your hamstrings as much as possible.*

Step 1: Begin this stretch in the deep squat rest position. Feet together. Hold your belly button area tight to your thighs. Firmly grasp your ankles and position your arms on the outside of the legs.

Step 2: Slowly extend your legs, trying to straighten them as much as possible. Do not allow your belly to come off of your thighs. Imagine that you are trying to hold a book in between.

Step 3: Hold this extension for anywhere from 1 second to 2 minutes. Return to deep squat rest position.

Step 4: Repeat this exercise as often as possible .

This is an uncomfortable stretch but one of the most beneficial in that into promotes a safer way to stretch the hamstrings without bending at the lumbar spine unnecessarily. The only joint that should be moving is your knee as you straighten your legs. When you find this exercise easier to perform, try it again but by placing both hands together flat on the floor in front of your feet in deep squat position. This will raise the difficulty but intensify the stretch.

*Tip: Maintain a straight back inline with your pelvis. Contract your abdominals and quadriceps in order to antagonize the resistance of the hamstrings. Avoid any conventional hamstring stretches that begin with a straight leg and requires that you bring your back to your legs for the movement.*

*Application: Tying shoelaces.*

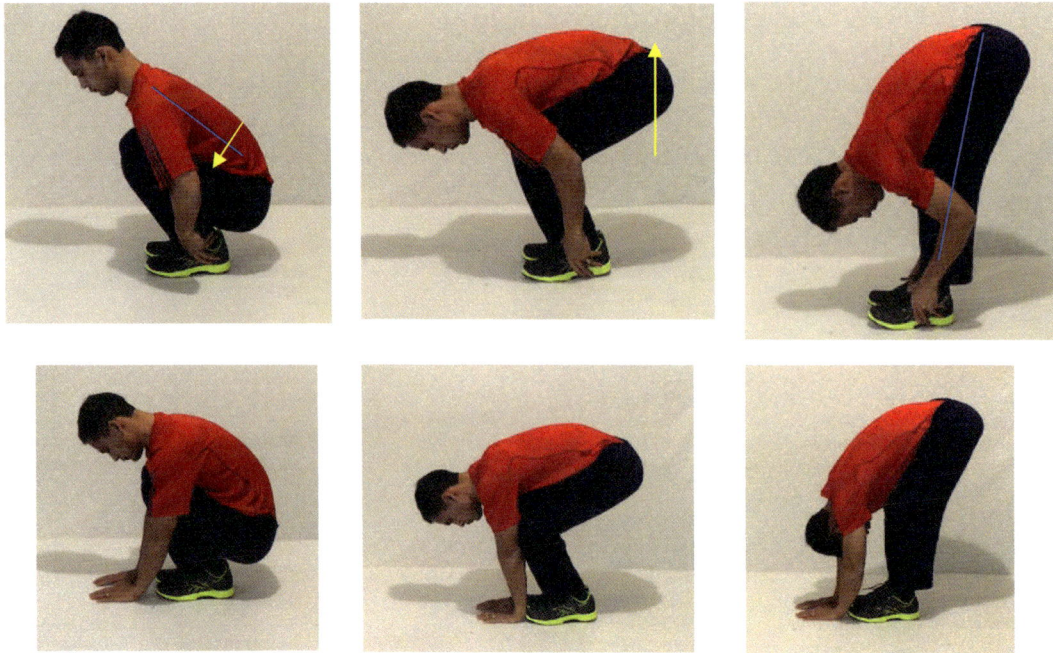

© 2014 SN Health Resources. Sherwin A. Nicholson.

## Squat (holds, leans, circles, steps, walks)

The are five variations and movements in this exercise. Altogether, this exercise will take time. You can perform them separately or together to increase the challenge. The purpose of this exercise is to condition your hips and back to be in this lowered stance and upright for long periods of time. By challenging the leg muscles, you can take much needed stress off of the back and support your back with minimal muscular exertion.

Begin this squat in any of three squat heights. Quarter squat (between full stance and half squat), half squat (thighs are horizontal) or deep squat (below horizontal but before resting on your ankles).

### Holds.

Step 1: Stand upright with feet shoulder width apart. Squat down to your desired squat height as mentioned above. Keep your back upright and arms out in front for balance. Do not allow your knees to lean forward past your toe line.

Step 2: Hold this position anywhere from 10 seconds to up to 2 minutes. Return to standing position to rest.

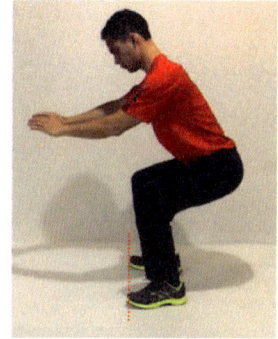

### Leans.

Step 3: Return to squat position and lean slightly forward by a few inches. Pause for 1-5 seconds, then return to original squat position. Next, lean to the right, back to centre, behind, back to center, and then to the left and back (clockwise). Return to standing to rest.

Step 4: Repeat in the other direction (counter clockwise).

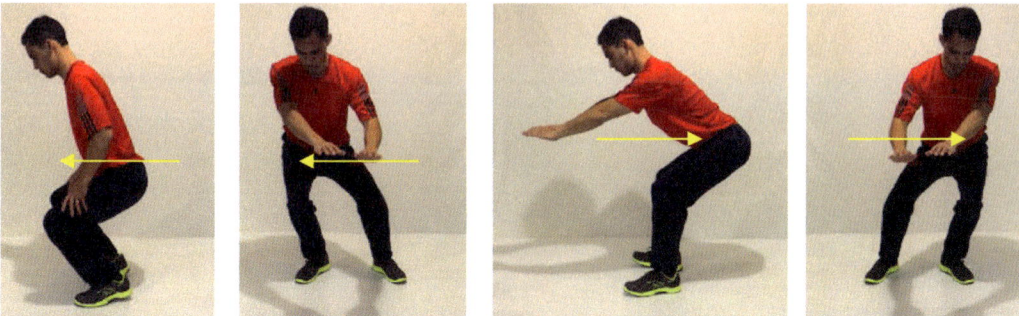

# Circles.

**Step 5:** Assume squat position. Circle your knees through the lean positions that you performed in step 3. Do not return to centre or pause but instead move continuously in a clockwise direction. Complete one full circle.

**Step 6:** Repeat the circle but in the other direction (counter clockwise). Return to rest position.

**Step 7:** Assume the squat position again. Slowly step forward about a half step each time. Bring the other foot forward also. Stay lowered, maintain squat height and a balanced posture.

**Step 8:** Step to the right sideways another half step with both feet. Then step backwards another half step. Then step sideways to the left with both feet until you reach the original standing spot. Stand to rest.

**Step 9:** Repeat in the other direction.

**Step 10:** Return to final squat position. Maintain height and posture. Face one direction at all times. Proceed to walk forward in half steps. After a few steps, step sideways to the right, then backwards, sideways to the left and back to original as before. Stand to rest.

**Step 11:** Repeat in the other direction.

*Tip: You can either place your hands on your hips if you prefer or out in front. You can also place them on your knees for support instead.*

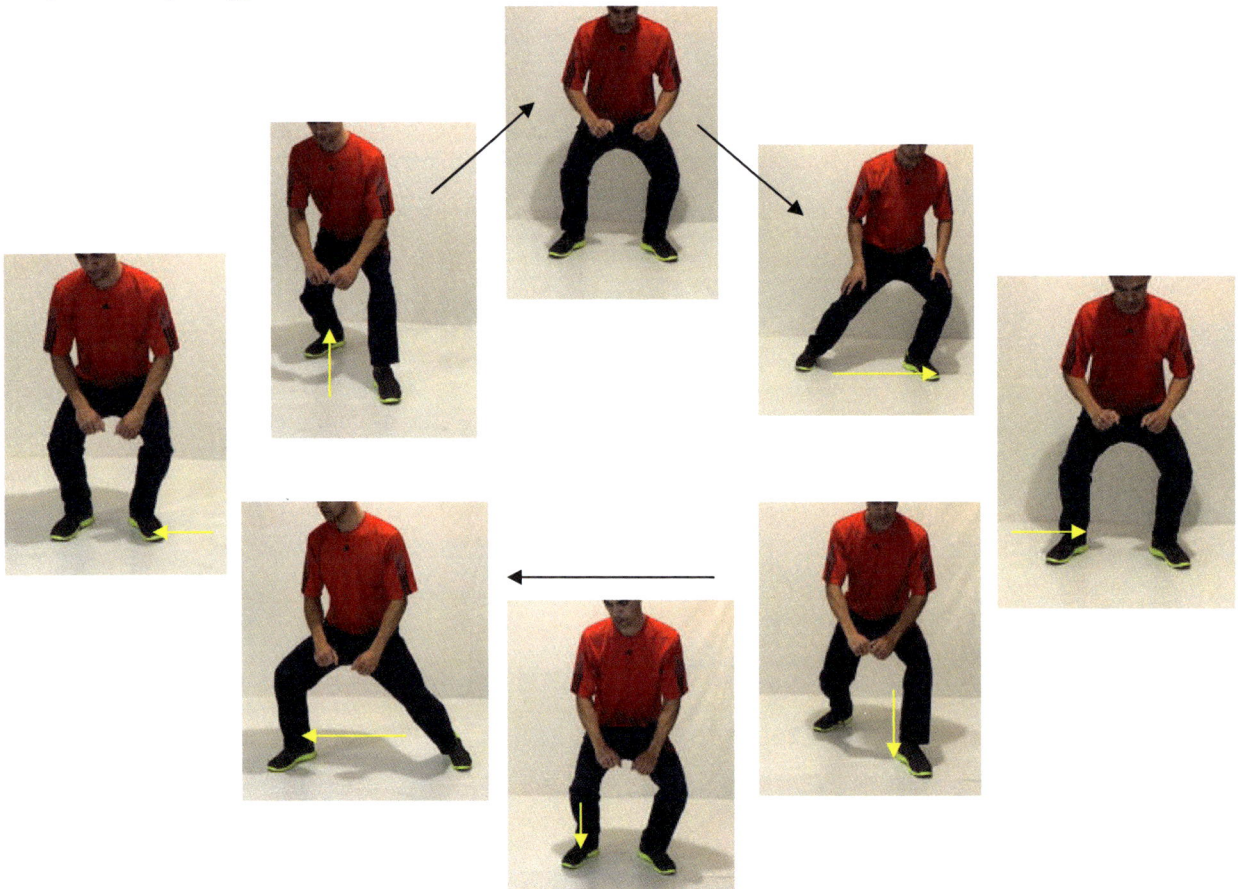

## Lunge with Reverse Kneel

This is a lunge with no assistance from your hands. Instead of lunging forward, perform this lunge backward. Keep your forward shin vertical and lower until your forward thigh is horizontal with the ground. Use a soft cushion for your knees. Maintain an upright posture. For balance, start with a support such as the back rest of a chair or a wall.

Step 1: Stand upright with your feet together. Position your arms for balance.

Step 2: Step backward a full step with your forward shin vertical. Bring the other leg straight backward until you can rest the knee to the ground gently.

Step 3: In this position, bring the forward leg back down and together with the other leg, placing both knees on the ground. Rest your buttocks on your legs and feet.

Step 4: Raise the other leg forward to a front lunge.

Step 5: Step forward using support from the arms and rear leg. Move back into the original squat position.

Step 6: Repeat this exercise but step backwards and alternate with the other leg instead.

Step 7: Repeat this entire exercise often.

*Tip: You can vary the amount in which you step backwards to alter the intensity of the exercise. Less is easier.*

*Application: Anytime that you need to lower yourself to the floor.*

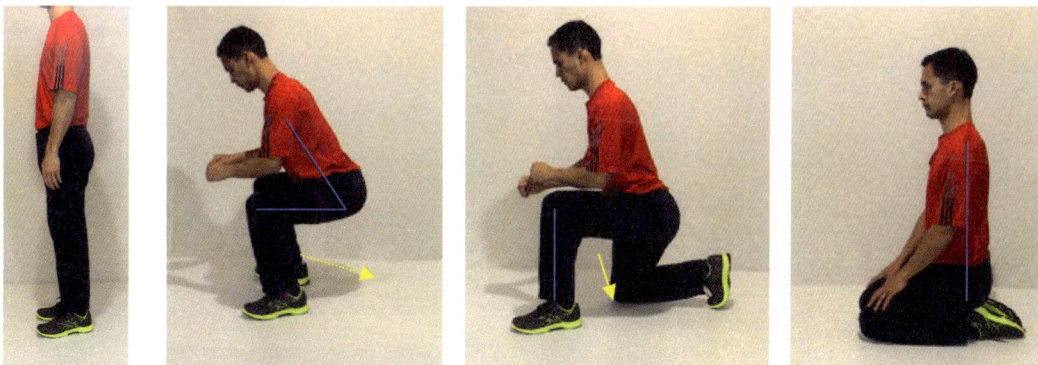

## Reverse Lunge

Reverse lunges are great for strengthening the entire lower body and training your hips to remain level. This exercise requires time to develop strength in the glutes and the quads. You should learn to perform this exercise slowly and to step backward into the lunge. Although lunge implies a forward movement, stepping backward activates your glutes easier than the forward method. You can choose to step forward after you have developed sufficient leg strength from the reverse lunge. Begin this exercise from the squat position and remain in this lowered position. *When you have mastered this exercise, you will be ready to perform the exercise from a standing position.*

Step 1: Lower your hips down into a squat position. Keep your feet shoulder width apart. Your thighs should be just above parallel to the floor. Place your hands on your hips.

Step 2: Bring one leg back until the thigh is vertical to the floor. Do not allow your knee to touch the floor. Use your hands on your hips to adjust and maintain your hips level and facing forward. Your back should be straight and upright.

Step 3: Hold this position for 1-10 seconds.

Step 4: Slowly bring your rear leg to the forward squat position. Keep your thigh parallel to the floor.

Step 5: Hold this position for 1-10 seconds.

Step 6: Return to a standing position and relax.

Step 7: Repeat often.

*Tip: If you contract your gluteus muscles before you step backward, it will improve their ability to activate at the right time during most activities.*

*Application: Anytime that you need to lower your body.*

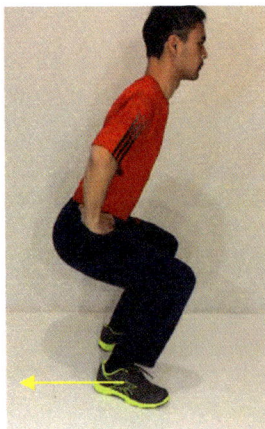

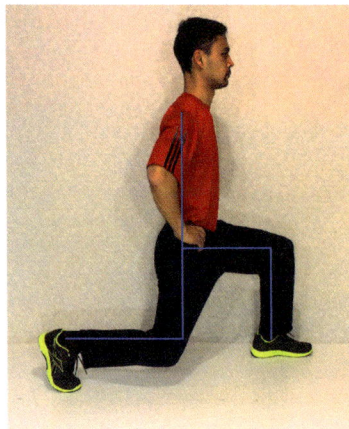

## Reverse Stair Step

This exercise helps to encourage the pelvis to tilt safely, mobilize the hips deeper and strengthen the gluteus muscles. It requires a step with handrails. Careful attention should be made as to avoid straining the knee. Do not allow your knee to bend and extend beyond your toe line. This will minimize any stress to the knee. As you step backward in this exercise, try to keep your shins vertical.

Step 1: Stand in front of a staircase with the back of your feet against the riser. Hold on to the rails for support.

Step 2: Raise one foot up and back to the first step. Try to keep your feet flat on both steps.

Step 3: Ease your body back until the raised shin and upper body is vertical.

Step 4: Contract your gluteus and thigh muscles to raise your body until your leg is straight again. Use the handrails for support.

Step 5: Repeat with the other leg.

Step 6: Try to reverse step up as many steps as comfortable with care to protect your knees.

*Tip: It is important to try to keep your hips level when you step upward and extend your leg. Practice your hip shift as you perform this exercise.*

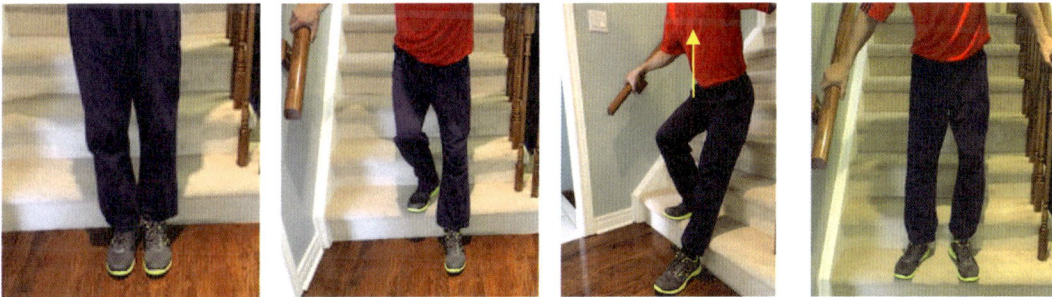

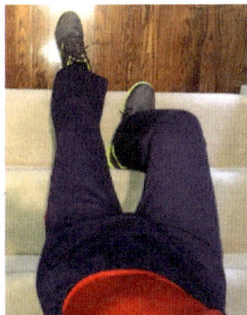

## Standing Knee to Chest (upright and leaning)

This is an exercise to strengthen the hip flexors in more than one position. It is meant to both strengthen and balance your legs at the same time. Without this type of balance, it is easy to suffer from back pain and disc issues. To perform this safely, you must be able to balance for a short period of time unassisted.

Step 1: Stand upright with feet together. Raise one leg up to a comfortable level and hold it up with your hands.

Step 2: Contract your hip muscles in order to keep your hips level with one another.

Step 3: Stay upright and hold for 10 seconds to 1 minute. Return to rest position.

Step 4: Repeat with the other leg.

Step 5: Perform this exercise, but this time with a forward lean.

During the forward lean, make sure that your spine is neutral and that your pelvis is in line with your lumbar spine. Allow your hamstrings to stretch and provide the tilt that you need. Do not bend at the spine. Make sure that your hips are level and avoid any hip dropping in this exercise.

*Application: Putting on socks, shoes, tying laces, etc...*

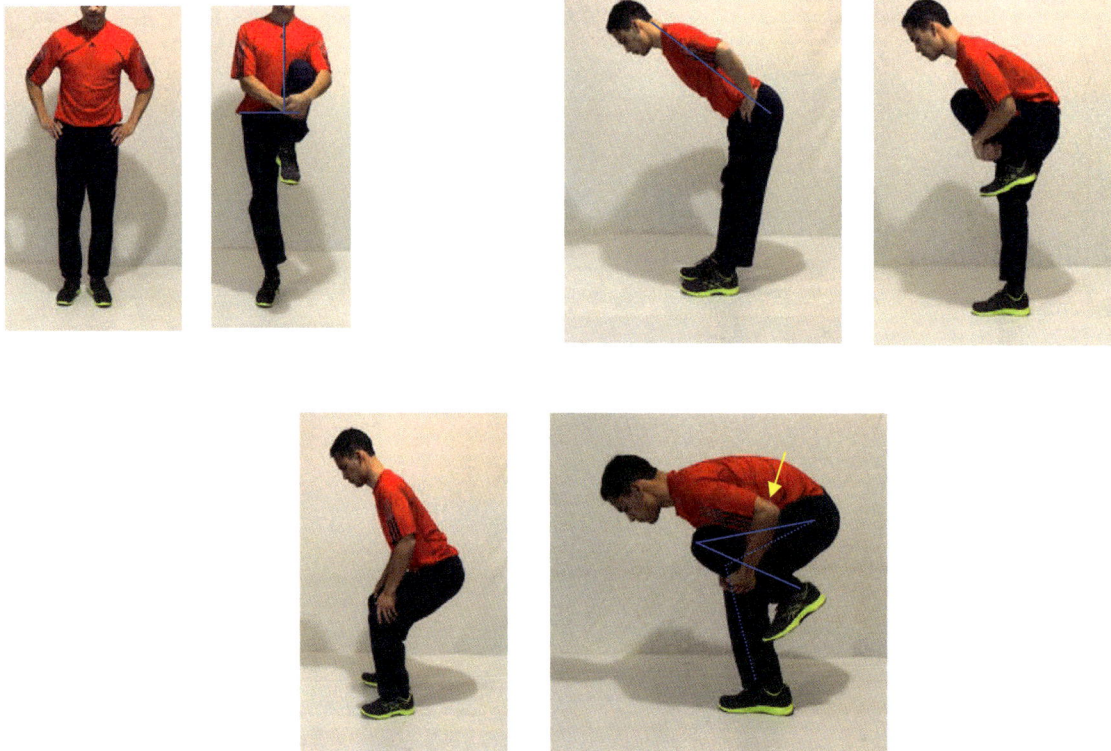

## Standing Hip Shift (leaning and bent knee)

This exercise is similar to the previous exercise but with added hip shifting.  It is more intense and requires that you maintain your balance for a longer period. When you perform this exercise,  it will be very challenging and there may be significant resistance to the movement and the tightness may still be present.

Step 1:  Stand upright, raise one leg and hold it up unassisted. Allow the unsupported hip to drop.

Step 2:  Raise the elevated and unsupported side of the hip by flexing the standing hip.  Raise in a slow controlled fashion as high as possible.   Your hip should be raised from below the level position to above level.

Step 3:  Hold the contraction and keep your hip raised for 1-10 seconds.

Step 4:  Return to a rest position.

Step 5:  Repeat with the other leg and hip.

Step 6:  Repeat this entire exercise but now with a forward lean.
Lean forward initially with a gentle lean while maintaining a neutral spine as mentioned in the previous exercise.  When you hold the upright position for a long enough time, the tension that resists will subside slowly and you will be able to continue to raise higher.
*Application:  Perform the leaning version when putting on socks, shoes and tying laces.*

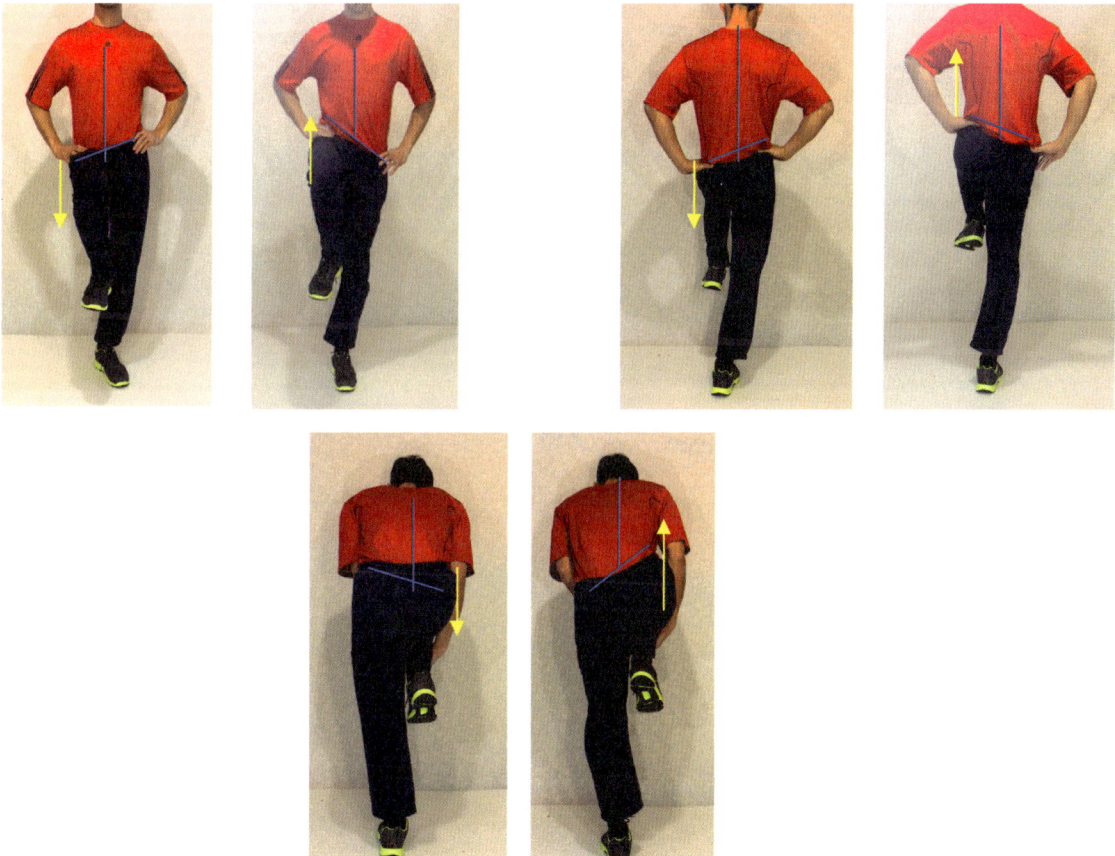

## Forward Stair Step with Hip Shift (assisted 2 riser)

Here, you can activate, strengthen your gluteus muscles, and strengthen your hips while in an upright position.  A staircase with handrail support is preferred as this exercise requires significant balance.

Step 1:  Stand in front of a staircase feet together while holding onto the handrail.

Step 2:  With one leg, step onto the second riser, raising your thigh to horizontal level or higher.  Contract your leg muscles to keep your hips level and horizontal.

Step 3: Raise up onto the second step while simultaneously, hip shifting the unsupported hip above the level of the other supported hip.  Maintain a vertical and neutral spine.   Keep your upper shin vertical.

Step 4:  Rest your upper foot on the second step after you have hip shifted fully.

Step 5:  Repeat with the other leg.

Step 5:  Go up as many steps as are available and come back down and repeat often.

*Application:  Perform this exercise whenever you travel upstairs.*

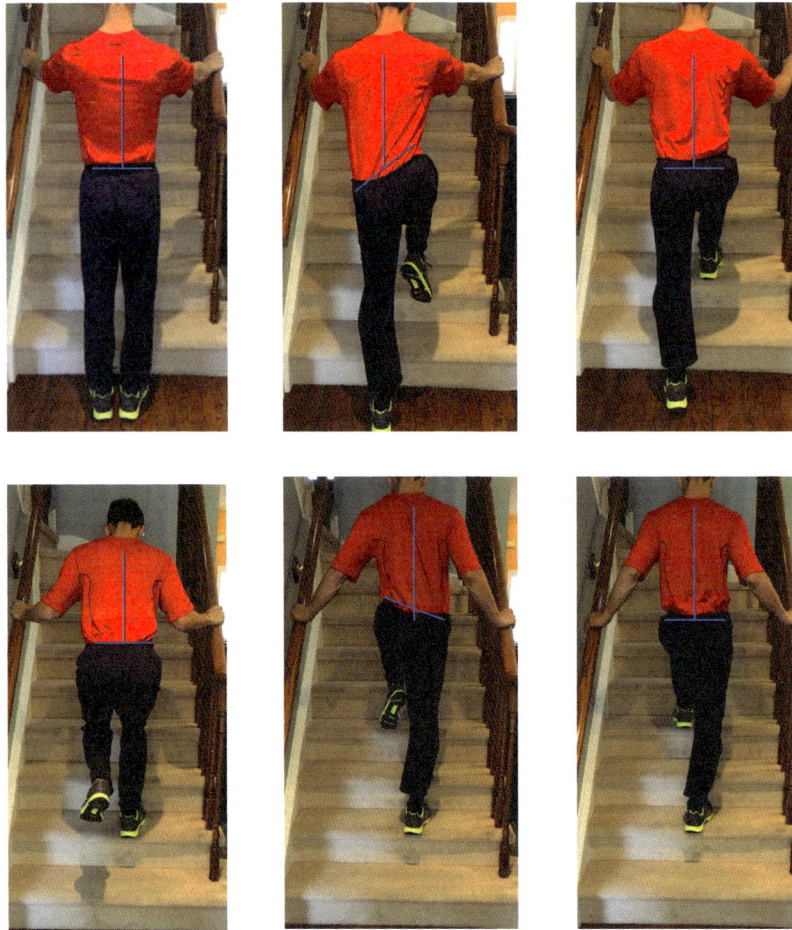

## Standing Leg Raise with Side Kick

With improved hip mobility and balance, you can use the strength developed in your hip muscles to maximize further hip mobility. Your will need a counter or a rail to help you with this exercise. Adjust the height of the counter or rail to be just under the level of your pelvis. Stand on a support for extra height if necessary.

Step 1: Stand in front of a counter with your back upright.

Step 2: Using your own balance if possible, raise your leg up above the level of the counter until you can extend it and straighten it out onto the counter. Bring your leg back down to the floor and rest.

Step 3: Repeat with the other leg.

Step 4: Turn your body sideways to the counter. Raise your leg until it is up above the level of the counter. Extend it and straighten it out sideways onto the counter. Rest and return your leg back down to the floor.

Step 5: Repeat with the other leg.

Step 6: Repeat this exercise as often as you can.

*Tip: Keep your supported leg flat on the floor. Use your arms to help you balance throughout this exercise. Try to begin this exercise with a fairly high counter or rail height and work your way up. Avoid leaning your upper body and maintain an upright posture as best as possible.*

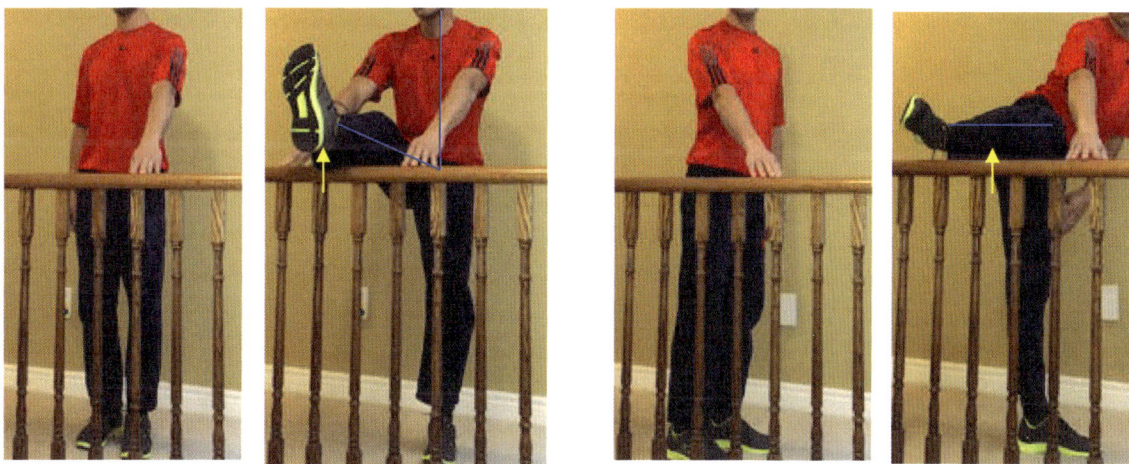

## Leg Flex (rail or counter)

This is a very advanced and difficult stretch. It will not be easy to perform at first but as you take your time with this exercise, your body will gradually relax into the hold that you are trying to make. By adding a twist, you can improve your back flexibility. Be very careful with your knee joint. Do not to apply excessive torque on it. Decrease the height of the counter or rail to reduce the amount of torque on your knee if necessary.

Step 1: Stand in front of a counter or a banister rail. Adjust the height to provide a sufficient challenge to the hips.
Keep your standing foot flat on the floor with the toes pointing out slightly. Grasp the counter or rail for balance.

Step 2: Raise, bend and rotate one leg up on to the counter with the inside shin facing the ceiling. Rest the foot and knee fully on the surface of the counter. The shin should be parallel to the counter or rail.

Step 3: Hold this position for 1 minute. Rest back down.

Step 4: Repeat with the other leg.

Step 5: Raise the original leg up again. Bend at the knee and rotate the leg so that the outside shin is now facing the ceiling. Rest this leg on the counter or rail. This shin should be parallel to the counter or rail as in step 2.

Step 6: Slowly twist your upper torso to grasp the foot of the raised leg with both hands.

Step 7: Hold this position for 1 minute. Rest back down.

Step 8: Repeat with the other leg.

Step 9: Repeat the entire exercise as often as needed in order to perform the exercise with little effort routinely.

Adding the twist makes the stretch harder but more effective at improving your lumbar flexibility. *As your flexibility improves, actively control the degree of the twist without using your hands, using only your back muscles.* Keep your lower foot flat on the ground to remain balanced. This stretch may initially tilt your pelvis sideways. As your body relaxes, the tilt will become less pronounced.

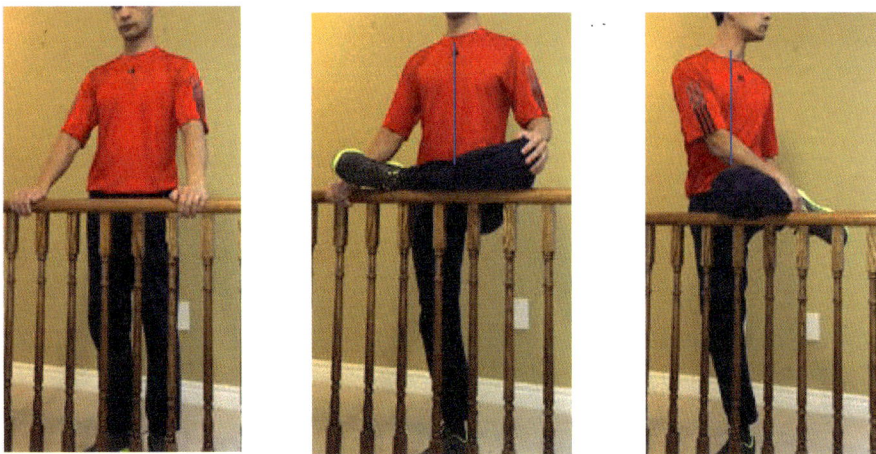

## Foot Raise (leaning and bent knee)

This is a very functional and practical exercise that you will find useful to perform during your daily dressing routine. It is also very challenging and requires advanced single leg balancing and leg strength.

Step 1: Stand with feet together and upright. Lean forward slightly with a neutral spine posture. Raise one knee fully up to your chest.

Step 2: Hold your hand out in front of the raised leg. Overlap the fingers tips of both hands.

Step 3: Slowly move your hands underneath your foot without touching the underside of your foot. Use your hip flexors or both sides of your hips to tilt the pelvis on an angle. The side of the pelvis with the raised foot should be higher than the side with the standing foot. Keep your abdominals contracted.

Step 4: Hold this position for 10 seconds to 1 full minute. Rest back down.

Step 5: Repeat with the other leg.

Step 6: Perform this entire exercise but begin with a half squat. Keep the half squat with the standing leg throughout the entire exercise.

Step 7: Repeat with the other leg.

Step 8: Perform the entire exercise from step 1 as often as is comfortable.

This exercise requires significant leg strength and balance in the squatting leg. It is more important to be balanced than to lift the foot above your fingers. To achieve both is desired though.

*Tip: Intensify this exercise by bending the standing leg as low as possible and then back up to straight. When you are ready, extend the length of time that you spend in the hold position to improve your conditioning.*

*Application: During your dressing routine, especially putting on and removing footwear and tying shoelaces.*

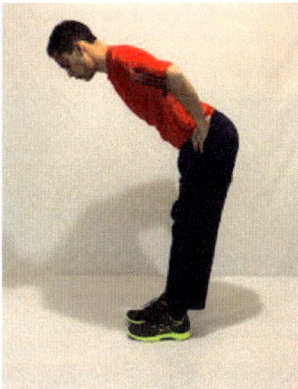

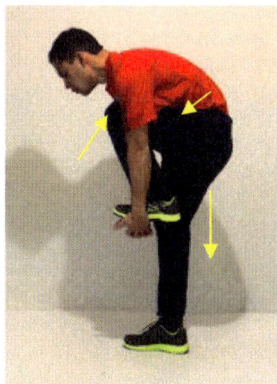

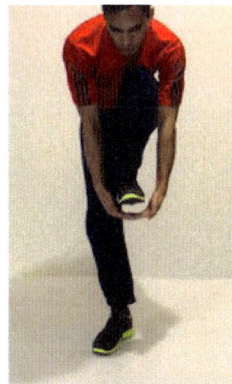

## Abdominal Leg Press

These abdominal exercises can be performed on any comfortable seat or floor. They will help to keep your lumbar curve neutral and counteract excessive anterior pelvic tilt. When you perform this exercise, maintain a neutral spine and avoid straining your neck. Use your arms and hands to stabilize your pelvic angle.

Step 1: Sit on the floor with your knees bent and together. Sit upright with a slightly flexed spine while using your arms to maintain this angle. Flex your toes.

Step 2: Contract your lower abdominal muscles and elevate your bent legs.

Step 3: Slowly slide your feet forward to full extension and then slide them in toward you fully without resting them on the floor.

Step 4: Perform this movement several times for as long as your stability and endurance permits.

*Tip: You can intensify this exercise by either elevating your legs higher, by moving them out and to the sides, or by pausing when you extend your legs.*

*Application: Before rising from bed and before lying into bed.*

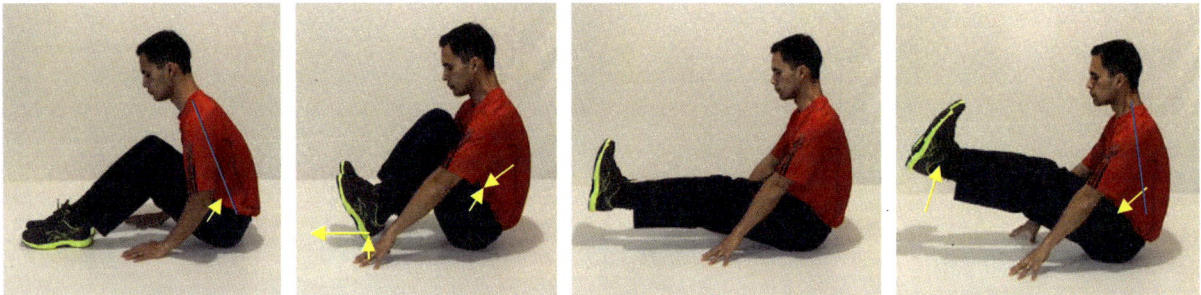

## Maintenance Exercises

Once you have mastered the Limited Mobility Exercises, made significant gains with the Progressive Exercises and are able to perform the Challenging Exercises with little difficulty, you can advance to the Maintenance Exercises.

The Maintenance Exercises will be all that you should need to perform on a regular basis to maintain a healthy spine and avoid unnecessary lower back pain. These exercises are the recommended ones but you can add any other exercise from the previous categories as needed or preferred.

All of these exercises are from the previous categories, with a focus on the Challenging Exercises. Perform these exercises as accurately as possible and with the same intensity. Lengthen the amount of time for each one to improve your conditioning. You will find that when you have mastered these exercises, you will not need to perform them as frequently as before; sometimes only weekly instead of daily.

1. Squat (walks)
2. Abdominal Leg Press
3. Seated Leg Rotation
4. Standing Abdominals
5. Plank with Steps
6. Lunge with Reverse Kneel
7. Foot Raise (leaning and bent knee)
8. Advanced Hamstring Stretch
9. Forward Stair Step with Hip Shift (assisted 2 riser)
10. Reverse Lunge
11. Seated Twist (unassisted)

The advantage of many of the maintenance and challenge exercises is that they are functional and practical. Therefore you can combine them with other natural movements that you can and should perform during your everyday routine. You may not feel that you are actually performing the exercise as it can blend in with your natural movements. These natural movements were once likely avoided due to back pain, but now they can be done with increased mobility, flexibility, strength and less pain.

## Supportive Exercises

These are recommended exercises that are to be performed as needed. They are standard, popular and not unique to the exercises designed for the Low Back Pain Program. They are very beneficial for relief from lower back pain.

Perform these exercises in a slow and controlled manner. Maintain a neutral spine with a safe pelvic tilt. Follow these exercises as recommended by an exercise class, personal trainer or other professional.

1. standing hamstring stretch
2. seated leg fold
3. side splits
4. side lean
5. lying rotator stretch
6. abdominal stretch (cobra)
7. floor hip stretch
8. buttock stretch (lying or standing)
9. balancing quad stretch
10. bridges

# Part Three - What to Use

## Progress Charts

These charts are meant to help you to keep track of the exercises as you complete them. They will help you to remember as there are too many to memorize. They are here for your reference especially when you are in the learning phase of the program.

Consider them 'completed' when you no longer find them difficult to perform and when you can perform them at length. The length refers to the number of repetitions and duration of time. There is no standard for number of repetitions and no fixed maximum time. The standard is your individual level of comfort. You can challenge yourself with your own length designations for the program.

The Maintenance Exercises chart has extra rows in which you can add your own exercises if preferred.

| Limited Mobility Exercises | Difficult | Difficult to Moderate | Moderate | Moderate to Easy | Easy |
|---|---|---|---|---|---|
| Deep Squat Rest | ■ | | ■ | | ■ |
| Kneeling Bow Rest | ■ | | ■ | | ■ |
| Seated Leg Opener | ■ | | ■ | | ■ |
| Seated Leg Rotation (assisted) | ■ | | ■ | | ■ |
| Seated Twist (assisted) | ■ | | ■ | | ■ |
| Seated Lunge | ■ | | ■ | | ■ |
| Leg Stretch (hamstrings and quads) | ■ | | ■ | | ■ |
| Calf Stretch | ■ | | ■ | | ■ |
| Hangs and Pushes | ■ | | ■ | | ■ |
| Lying Twist | ■ | | ■ | | ■ |
| Abdominal Crunch | ■ | | ■ | | ■ |
| Quadriceps Stretch | ■ | | ■ | | ■ |
| Seated Knee Raise | ■ | | ■ | | ■ |

| Progressive Exercises | Difficult | Difficult to Moderate | Moderate | Moderate to Easy | Easy |
|---|---|---|---|---|---|
| Seated Hip Adjustment (assisted) | ■ | | ■ | | ■ |
| Seated and Floor Hip Shift | ■ | | ■ | | ■ |
| Seated Leg Rotation (assisted with contraction) | ■ | | ■ | | ■ |
| Seated Leg Cross with Forward Lean | ■ | | ■ | | ■ |
| Floor Leg Bend and Shift | ■ | | ■ | | ■ |
| Seated Leg to Chest | ■ | | ■ | | ■ |
| Leaning Hip Shift | ■ | | ■ | | ■ |
| Rail Squat (assisted) | ■ | | ■ | | ■ |
| Seated Hamstring Stretch (in and out) | ■ | | ■ | | ■ |
| Stair Step (up and down) | ■ | | ■ | | ■ |
| Reverse Stair Squat Lean | ■ | | ■ | | ■ |
| Hip Opener (inside and outside) | ■ | | ■ | | ■ |
| Seated Calf Stretch | ■ | | ■ | | ■ |
| Double Leg Rotation | ■ | | ■ | | ■ |
| Deep Abdominal Crunch (leg raised) | ■ | | ■ | | ■ |
| Plank with Steps | ■ | | ■ | | ■ |
| Couch Split | ■ | | ■ | | ■ |
| Outside Hip Stretch | ■ | | ■ | | ■ |
| Standing Abdominal | ■ | | ■ | | ■ |

| Challenging Exercises | Difficult | Difficult to Moderate | Moderate | Moderate to Easy | Easy |
|---|---|---|---|---|---|
| Seated Leg Lift (multidirectional) | ■ | | ■ | | ■ |
| Advanced Hamstring Stretch (ankle and floor) | ■ | | ■ | | ■ |
| Squat (holds, leans, circles, steps, walks) | ■ | | ■ | | ■ |
| Lunge with Reverse Kneel | ■ | | ■ | | ■ |
| Reverse Lunge | ■ | | ■ | | ■ |
| Reverse Stair Step | ■ | | ■ | | ■ |
| Sanding Knee to Chest (upright and leaning) | ■ | | ■ | | ■ |
| Standing Hip Shift (leaning and bent knee) | ■ | | ■ | | ■ |
| Forward Stair Step with Hip Shift (assisted 2 riser) | ■ | | ■ | | ■ |
| Standing Leg Raise with Side Kick | ■ | | ■ | | ■ |
| Leg Flex (rail or counter) | ■ | | ■ | | ■ |
| Foot Raise (lean and bend) | ■ | | ■ | | ■ |
| Abdominal Leg Press | ■ | | ■ | | ■ |

| Maintenance Exercises | Difficult | Difficult to Moderate | Moderate | Moderate to Easy | Easy |
|---|---|---|---|---|---|
| Squat (walks) | | | | | |
| Abdominal Leg Press | | | | | |
| Seated Leg Rotation | | | | | |
| Standing Abdominals | | | | | |
| Plank with Steps | | | | | |
| Lunge with Reverse Kneel | | | | | |
| Foot Raise (leaning and bent knee) | | | | | |
| Advanced Hamstring Stretch | | | | | |
| Forward Stair Step with Hip Shift (2 riser) | | | | | |
| Reverse Lunge | | | | | |
| Seated Twist (unassisted) | | | | | |
| | | | | | |
| | | | | | |
| | | | | | |

# Additional Help

At this point, you have a much better understanding and awareness of the exercises and movements that you need to perform in order to prevent and reduce lower back pain.

You should be able to move and position yourself differently than you have before beginning this program. Consider that these exercises are not simply to be used outside of your regular daily activity but are to be incorporated within your day-to-day routines.

Keep aware of which exercises and movements that you can blend together with simple tasks that you perform during your waking hours. These tasks range from getting dressed, carrying and lifting objects to bending and squatting down to perform a chore. You will find it very easy to use these exercises everyday as they are functional and practical.

This is the advantage of the program. Although it is a very challenging and lengthy one, it can gradually minimize itself to basic movements in your daily routines. It should not have to feel like you are performing a separate workout or exercise program. Rather, it should be more of a conditioning program to get you back to the movements that your body requires to function effectively and efficiently everyday.

The only concern with this program may be the amount of time required to perform and accomplish the exercises within it in order to achieve long term low back pain relief.

You should now have a stronger, more flexible and stable body. It will give you proper mobility and protect your lower spine, provided that you follow the program as directed. You should also be able to move differently and safer than before with respect to your lower back.

Lower back pain is very complex, but a good program can offer protection from it. If you follow the program but you are still affected by lower back pain, consider that there may be other contributing factors that are beyond the scope of this program. Please continue to seek further professional help and never give up on finding the proper treatment for your low back pain.

I sincerely thank you for using the program and wish you lasting relief and a more enjoyable lifestyle.

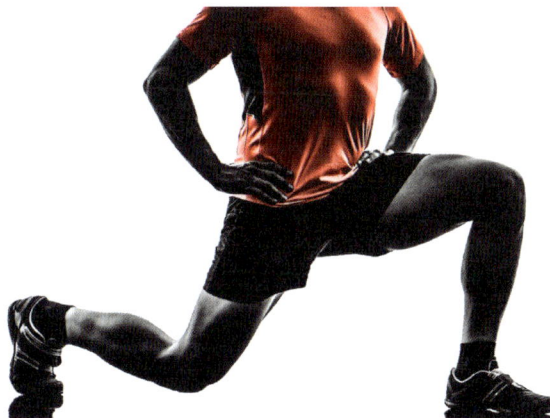

Notes:

Tennis Pathways Ltd
48195560
30 97 41
Navel gp m 4.38

Printed in Great Britain
by Amazon